To Jeffrey North

The
American Way
of Life
Need Not Be
Hazardous to Your
Health

30th Birthday from his
mother and Father who
hope the suggestions herein
and his own good sense
will enable him to enjoy
many happy returns.

The American Way of Life Need Not Be Hazardous to Your Health

REVISED EDITION

JOHN W. FARQUHAR, M.D.

ADDISON-WESLEY PUBLISHING COMPANY, INC.
Reading, Massachusetts   Menlo Park, California   New York
Don Mills, Ontario   Wokingham, England   Amsterdam   Bonn
Sydney   Singapore   Tokyo   Madrid   San Juan

For a complete listing of sources for figures and tables, please see p. 199.

Library of Congress Cataloging-in-Publication Data

Farquhar, John W., 1927–
   The American way of life need not be hazardous to your
health.

   Bibliography: p.
   Includes index.
   1. Health.   2. Cardiovascular system—Diseases—
Prevention—Popular works.   3. Behavior modification.
I. Title.   [DNLM: 1. Cardiovascular Diseases—prevention &
control—popular works.   2. Health Promotion—popular
works.   3. Life Style—popular works.   4. Self Care—
popular works.   WA 590 F238a]
RA776.5.F34   1987   616.1'05   87–12654
ISBN 0–201–12186–7 (pbk.)

Cover design by Victoria Blaine
Text design by Stanford Alumni Association
Set in 11-point Palatino by Harrison Typesetting, Inc., Portland, OR

CDEFGHIJ-DO-898
Third Printing, September 1988

This book was published originally as a part of the Portable Stanford, a
book series published by the Stanford Alumni Association, Stanford,
California.

To Christine, Meg, and Jolly,
who made it all possible.

CONTENTS

ACKNOWLEDGMENTS

I am indebted to many of my colleagues in the interdisciplinary Stanford Center for Research in Disease Prevention for their roles in critiquing and commenting upon this manuscript in its various stages. Dr. Carl Thoresen was particularly influential in directing my approach to teaching methods for achieving self-directed change. I am also grateful to Drs. Brian Danaher, Stephen Fortmann, William Haskell, C. Barr Taylor, and Peter Wood, all of whom generously gave their time and expertise, providing valuable appraisals of the manuscript. In addition, Prudence Breitrose furnished helpful comments and suggestions for changes. Drs. Albert Bandura and Nathan Maccoby of Stanford University, Dr. Henry Blackburn of the University of Minnesota, and Dr. William Connor of the University of Oregon deserve special mention for their many formative influences in furthering my understanding of the subjects treated in this book.

With my deepest gratitude and respect, I wish to thank my editor for the first edition, Cynthia Fry Gunn, who encouraged me through many difficult hours with her imperturbable patience and good cheer.

Dr. Alvin Tarlov, President of the Kaiser Family Foundation, was influential in providing concepts useful in preparing the second edition. My colleague, Dr. Gene Spiller, was particularly helpful in creating an updated second edition. My secretary, Sydney Ludowese, has my gratitude for her able support. Finally, I wish to thank the many members and friends of the Stanford Center for

Research in Disease Prevention, too numerous to mention individually, for their interest, participation, and enthusiastic support which have made the program such a success.

I claim responsibility for all errors and omissions.

John W. Farquhar

INTRODUCTION TO THE REVISED EDITION

As I prepare the second edition of this book, the awareness of the need for prevention of non-infectious chronic diseases has reached an all-time high. Disease prevention has emerged in the 1980s as a greater national priority than ever before. The $50 million federal allotment in 1978, the date of the first edition of this book, rose to $3 billion in 1984, and many government organizations have become deeply involved in these efforts.

The recent efforts at partial repair, such as coronary artery bypass surgery, constitute a pure growth industry: In 1971 only 10,000 such operations were performed; in 1977 there were about 70,000, and the figure has since climbed to over 170,000 each year, at a cost of over $2 billion a year. Unfortunately, this procedure does not insure permanent health. Often the surgery must be repeated after a few years. Since 1980 another new growth industry has sprung up, "balloon angioplasty," a less expensive alternative to bypass grafts. Unfortunately, however, the narrowed artery now opened by the high pressure balloon has a strong tendency to close down again.

Given the cost and failure rate of these methods, it is inevitable that society will increasingly question the wisdom of total obeisance to the route of post-symptomatic repair. Ill health is not an isolated event; it is the result of an accumulation of abuses, each seemingly inconsequential. Eventually they take their toll. I believe that the individual has to accept responsibility for maintaining his or her own health. No one else can—not a doctor, not a fleet of doctors. In the way we live our daily lives, we either enhance our health or diminish it.

Often we assume that our life-style is healthy, that everything is "normal," when in fact we are following a path inimical to our health. I hear people say, "I really should lose weight," or "I ought to get more exercise," or "I know I should quit smoking." Yet, free to choose, we often continue along the same hazardous course, living as if our lives were charmed—"It won't happen to me." Our lives are not charmed; rather than forfeit our birthright of good health, we should protect it.

The overwhelming majority of fatal and near-fatal episodes of premature heart attack and stroke are preventable, as are, in all probability, a large percentage of cases of adult-onset diabetes, osteoporosis, and diet-related cancers. This book contains in one volume information on all health habits that are associated with heart attacks, strokes, and other chronic diseases and provides practical, self-directed methods for lowering your risk level in each of these areas. As you read the chapters that follow—on chronic disease, risk assessment, methods of self-directed change, stress management, exercise, nutrition and food patterns, weight control, and smoking— you will see how one aspect of your health affects other aspects as well, and how the prevention of one disease is often the prevention of many diseases. To receive maximum benefit, I suggest that you read the chapters in sequence.

Much of medicine needs to be demystified: For this to happen, high-quality health education is vital. It is my deepest hope that someday the quality of public health education will be so high, and our society so supportive of healthful life-styles, that we will find it simple to retain our natural birthright of good health. Until that time, this book is one man's attempt to work toward that goal. I undertake here to discuss not only what I believe you should know about preventable risks for heart disease, stroke, certain common cancers, and diabetes but also what you can do to bring about permanent life-enhancing changes that will reduce these risks.

We were born healthy and we can die healthy when our days run out. We can keep our lungs clean and our arteries free of plaque as easily as we can keep our minds full of good hope. Why cannot we as a nation reclaim the gift we were given at birth—good health and vigorous bodies—and stand up against passivity? Let us be in charge of how we live by showing resistance to the quick fixes of modernity. Let us reach out and take what is naturally ours. Let us, for the first time ever, combine true prevention with wise thinking.

John W. Farquhar, M.D.

Stanford, California, 1987

1

THE AMERICAN WAY OF LIFE

I lost a friend yesterday. Death set upon him like a monster, gripping him with pain and fear, overwhelming him with fatigue, and finally shaking him loose, lifeless. Gone is a husband, gone a father, gone a brother. In my grief, I am angry. Death came early, uninvited; it was not a welcome release at the end of a fulfilled life. It came as an interloper, seizing a man at the center of his time.

On a Sunday five months ago at around bedtime, Roger complained of indigestion to his wife, Ellen. He had eaten nothing out of the ordinary for dinner—meat, potatoes, vegetables, some cheesecake left over from a party the night before. He lay down, tried to concentrate on the 10 o'clock news on television, asked his wife to get him a bicarbonate of soda. They switched on a late movie and she fell asleep. At two in the morning Roger telephoned me.

What impressed me immediately, and what I remember so clearly now, were not his words but his voice. It was small, fearful, astonished. He clearly knew what was happening to him. He said the pain was now in his lower chest; he was sweating heavily; he felt very weak. Then he passed the telephone to Ellen. I told her I would call for an ambulance and meet them at the hospital. I dressed and rushed over to the coronary care unit at Stanford Hospital.

Roger was wheeled into the hospital in shock. Ellen, behind him, was extraordinarily calm. Diagnosis confirmed that a major coronary thrombosis had occurred.

At this point, high technology took over. All vital functions were continuously monitored and Roger's wounded heart muscle was gently prodded and shaped into a force that could just barely sustain life. Roger was not fully alert or aware of the drama and tension around him. He did not know that the many highly trained health professionals working swiftly about him were processing yet another common entrant into a tunnel from which it can be predicted that only one in four, given his state of shock on entry, would emerge alive at the end of a week.

The initial fear Roger felt, along with his crisis of pain, became the fear of his friends, his family, and those of us who were caring for him. We watched him return to awareness 48 hours after the attack. At this point, Roger had, statistically speaking, passed his first hurdle and thus increased his chances for surviving a week to one in two.

Three weeks after his attack, tubes for intravenous feeding were removed and continuous monitoring ended. Roger was transferred from the fury and precarious balance of the coronary care unit to a quiet ward. His wife's fears eased. In another two weeks, still with a fragile hold on life, Roger was allowed to go home.

To Roger, home meant the comfort and security of his family and his own surroundings. To his family, having Roger home meant adjusting to his needs, watching him regain some of his strength, seeing him occasionally cry. His children had not quite realized how near death he had been. He was still profoundly exhausted and had recurrent sensations of irregular heart poundings. He was bewildered and depressed. He relied on his wife to assist with his frequent medications.

In the three months following his heart attack, Roger re-entered the hospital twice for brief treatments for shortness of breath due to a weakened heart. He also entered a new statistical group: He was now one in two to survive three months. Over the next four weeks his condition stabilized slightly. Even though he was virtually bedridden, Roger and his family maintained their constant hope and belief that life would eventually return to normal.

One afternoon a few weeks later, Ellen came home from grocery shopping and found Roger in immense pain. She drove him directly to the hospital. The chest pain continued for hours; then suddenly it was over. Roger died.

From the time of his initial heart attack until his death, Roger suffered greatly. Even the simplest exertion, such as walking to the bathroom, caused shortness of breath. His ankles were so swollen that he had to wear support bandages. He ate little. He lost interest in sex. Depression was a continuing problem. He frequently awoke in the night and sat on the edge of the bed gasping for air. These episodes, along with the strange poundings in his chest, created an atmosphere of unspoken anxiety and uncertainty in the family.

HEART DISEASE TODAY

Medical records tell us when Roger experienced his first myocardial infarction (the medical term for a serious heart attack in which an already narrowed artery is blocked and damage to a part of the heart muscle then occurs), and they tell us when he died. But they do not tell us when in Roger's 48 years of life he embarked on a path that led him to premature death.

When was the first hint that he had slipped across the line into a special group of about 248,000 Americans under age 75 who each year die prematurely from heart attacks? Had Roger been luckier, he might have belonged to another group of 600,000 who suffer heart attacks that are not fatal. (These survivors, however, have a high risk of future fatal heart attacks.) Every year an additional 236,000 Americans under age 75 have strokes, 52,000 of which are fatal. Both heart attacks and strokes are due almost entirely to a process called *atherosclerosis*, in which arteries to the brain, heart, and other organs become progressively narrowed by deposits of cholesterol and fibrous tissue.

The dream of an abundant, full life dissolves for all, like Roger, who die prematurely. If we use 75 as the age before which death is defined as premature, heart attack is the largest single cause of premature death in the United States. We are still in the midst of a modern epidemic of heart disease. At least 90 percent of the fatal and near-fatal episodes of premature strokes and heart attacks are preventable. This is truly a staggering percentage, and it carries a vital message to virtually everyone. By the way you live, you greatly determine not only the length of your life but also the quality of your life.

Millions of us have learned that lesson. In the past decade, medical scientists, the media, and the climate of the times have all combined to induce changes in the way we live on a truly encouraging scale. These changes, including a significant drop in cigarette smoking, are very likely responsible for the surprising fact that the heart attack rate has been *decreasing* recently—down 36 percent since the peak of the epidemic in 1965. Much can be done to accelerate this reduction; the best estimate is that we can further reduce the death rate from heart attack to one-tenth or less of its 1965 peak. The journey will be long and slow for the nation at large; the arrival time will depend on the rate of adoption of healthier life-styles and creation of healthy environments by American society.

HABITS AND LIFE-STYLE

What this book discusses applies to all aspects of our lives—what we eat, how we exercise, how we deal with daily stresses. How we handle these aspects to a large degree dictates our physical and mental well-being. What we are today is the aggregate of genetic factors, the influences of early experiences and learning, and personal habits concerning diet, exercise, smoking, and stress, which constitute our life-style.

What is the impact of our life-patterns on our national health? To the annual total in 1982 of 248,000 premature deaths from heart attacks and strokes, we must add the total impact of cigarette smoking on our health. This includes 90,000 fatalities from lung cancer, about 20,000 fatalities from other types of cancer, 46,000 deaths from emphysema and other chronic lung problems. In addition, we must include about one million individuals who currently suffer from significant degrees of pulmonary crippling. There is also impressive and growing evidence that the incidence of cancer of the breast, colon, and rectum is increased by certain longstanding dietary practices (to be discussed in a later chapter). Therefore, another group of cancers can be added to the list of health problems partly preventable through modified dietary habits, and more than one-third of all cancers are now considered to be diet-related.

ONE MAN'S LIFE-SHORTENING PATH

Early Eating Habits and Cholesterol

From this larger perspective, let us return to Roger's particular case. The shortening of Roger's life began long before his initial heart attack. At birth, Roger was a perfectly healthy baby—well-formed, strong, and vigorous. Roger's mother was concerned that the family's diet be a good one. As Roger was growing up, there was great emphasis on providing adequate protein. Thus, Roger's early childhood diet included an excessive representation of eggs, cheese, whole milk, meat, ice cream, and butter—believed to be healthful and high in needed protein and calcium for a growing child. This is also a high-cholesterol and high-saturated-fat diet, full of foods that tend to increase deposits of fat in the arteries.

The importance of early childhood diet on blood cholesterol—one of the three major risk factors in heart disease, along with smoking and the level of blood pressure—is demonstrated by Figure 1-1. The levels of blood cholesterol in a group of schoolchildren in Wisconsin were compared to the levels in a group of healthy schoolchildren living in a rural mountain village in Mexico. The Wisconsin children had an average blood cholesterol level of 187, whereas the Mexican children had an average blood cholesterol level of 97—about half that of the Wisconsin children. It is important to note that each group showed a wide range of cholesterol levels (due largely to hereditary factors). What is even more significant is that the blood cholesterol levels of the Mexican children were so much lower that very little overlap existed between the two groups, despite the wide range of levels. This separation between the groups indicates that *between* cultures environmental factors are more important determinants of blood cholesterol levels than are genetic factors; however, *within* any one culture genetic factors are the dominant influence.

The difference in blood cholesterol levels between the Mexican and Wisconsin children was attributed largely to the higher intake of

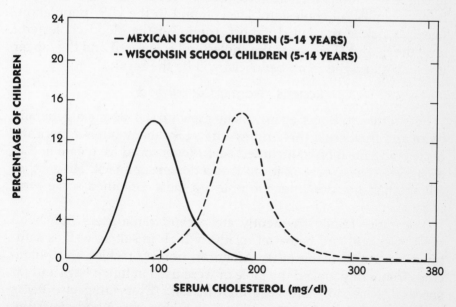

Figure 1-1: Graph showing wide differences in blood cholesterol levels of Mexican and Wisconsin children.

dietary cholesterol and dietary saturated fat from eggs, meat, milk, and cheese by the Wisconsin children. In addition to eating foods low in saturated fat, the Mexican children exercised more, which made them leaner and may also have contributed to the difference in cholesterol levels. Similarly, the Mexican children consumed greater amounts of dietary fiber. This fiber intake or perhaps other dietary factors that we do not yet understand may have helped, too, in keeping the Mexican children's cholesterol levels low.

Studies such as these lead us to believe that the risk factors for atherosclerosis begin in early childhood and develop over many years. These facts also suggest that public health efforts should be directed at the entire population (rather than merely to those in the highest risk categories) in order to lower risk-factor levels in all people and at all ages. Were we to treat only the most risk-prone group—those having special genetic factors that separate them from the majority—we would be ignoring countless individuals who pursue habits that subject them to needless risk. We would be overlooking the fact that body weight, blood cholesterol, and blood pressure tend to increase with age among the so-called normal population in the United States; we would therefore miss our opportunity to prevent problems before they develop. Cardiovascular risk increases in concert with blood cholesterol over a wide range of levels; therefore, at almost all cholesterol levels found in the U.S. population, needless risk is present. In short, the lower the blood cholesterol level the better. The sooner the cholesterol is lowered and the longer it remains low, the more beneficial will be the results.

Roger's "Normal" Childhood

Let's return to Roger again. As he grew up, he ate meat generally twice and frequently three times a day. Like many other Americans his evening meal often included beef. Roger loved ice cream and at least five times a week enjoyed it as a dessert or snack. His mother felt she had not done her job unless a meal contained some form of meat.

The entire family frequently ate bacon, frankfurters, luncheon meat, sausage, and ham—all relatively high in salt as well as saturated fat. As in many other American homes, pickles and potato chips frequently graced the table or were used in lunch bags and for snacks. These, too, are very high in salt. (Everything else being equal, the higher the salt intake the higher the blood pressure. Again, as with levels of blood cholesterol and the intake of choles-

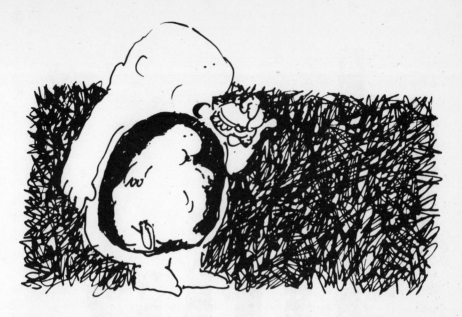

terol and saturated fat, so it is with blood pressure and salt intake: Genetically determined susceptibility affects the response to the dietary factors. Hence, while virtually all people will have a blood pressure rise with increased salt intake, those who are genetically more susceptible will have greater blood pressure increases.)

Not only was Roger a plump baby (which Roger's parents regarded as fine—just "baby fat"), he was also a chubby child. Snacks were provided as pacifiers and as rewards for good behavior. His family environment included easy access to the cookie jar, candy treats, and open bowls of snack foods. Such ready access to sugary snacks created habits that contributed to Roger's weight gain. These habits were difficult to reverse in adult life. Roger was not considered obese, but throughout his childhood he was in the top third of his age group in terms of weight.

According to numerous studies, Americans lead the world in their average degree of overweight. Figure 1-2 (next page) shows the percent of a sample of Americans (males 40-59) considered to be overweight on the basis of their skinfold thickness (which measures the depth of the fat layer) compared to samples of males from six other countries. Again, everything else being equal, the heavier one is, the higher the blood pressure and the higher the amount of cholesterol in the blood. The influence of weight gain or loss is, however, stronger on blood pressure level than it is on cholesterol level.

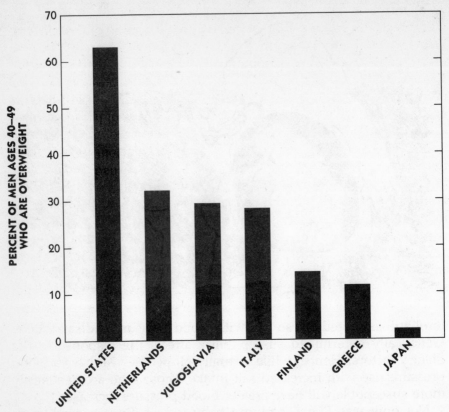

Figure 1-2: Comparison of degree of overweight in males aged 40-59 in population samples of seven countries.

Now we can understand that Roger's "normal" weight of a few extra pounds and his "normal" diet, which was rich in calories, sugar, salt, cholesterol, and saturated fat, worked together over time to raise his body weight and his blood pressure and blood cholesterol levels to unhealthy heights.

The Slow Road to Cardiovascular Disease

In much of the modern Western world, including the United States, a gradual increase in blood pressure and blood cholesterol is accepted as a "normal" accompaniment of age. These increases typically do not occur in primitive societies. Once primitive societies come into contact with modern civilization, however, such increases often do occur. A study of five tribes in the Solomon Islands by Dr. Lot Page of Harvard and his associates showed that the degree of increase in blood pressure was correlated with the degree of acculturation, that is, adoption of dietary and occupational practices of Western man. It was significant that the introduction of "tinned meat" (high in salt) was accompanied by a rise in blood pressure. The investigators also noticed an increase in body weight that occurred in conjunction with changes in eating and exercise habits, and this was associated with further increases in blood pressure.

Coronary arteries are the first to be choked off by cholesterol deposits (probably because of the greater turbulence of blood flow that makes the inner lining of these arteries more sensitive to the injurious effects of high blood cholesterol and blood pressure). They are the only source of blood to the heart, which cannot tolerate as much arterial narrowing and the resulting reduction in oxygen as can, for example, the legs or abdominal organs.

Evidence that damage to the coronary arteries is present even in early adulthood is illustrated most strikingly by a study of American soldiers killed in action during the Korean War. It was discovered that 35 percent of these American soldiers (whose average age was 22) had greater than 15 percent narrowing of their coronary arteries due to abnormal collections of cholesterol. These deposits are almost never found in young Koreans or in young adults of other countries whose populations share similarly low blood cholesterol levels. (The average cholesterol level of adults in Japan—where the diet is low in saturated fat and cholesterol and similar to that of Korea—is about 140 milligrams per deciliter, 33 percent lower than that of adults in the United States.)

Figure 1-3 (next page) compares the cholesterol levels found in 1965 among men aged 40 to 59 in two areas of southern Japan and an area of eastern Finland. At that time Finland had a higher heart attack rate than any other country in the world, and also the highest cholesterol levels—considerably higher than Americans. Dr. Ancel Keys, a cardiovascular disease epidemiologist, and his co-workers attribute the Finnish cholesterol levels to intakes of cheese, butter, and milk believed to be among the highest in the world. This high butterfat intake is added to the so-called normal level of meat and egg intake characteristic of the rest of the Western world. Since the studies of Dr. Keys, the Finnish government has succeeded in lowering butterfat intake, and the cholesterol levels and heart attack rates of the Finnish people have dropped.

Work done by Dr. Keys and his co-workers showed a surprisingly strong correlation of heart attack rates with the cholesterol levels in seven countries selected for study. They also found that an

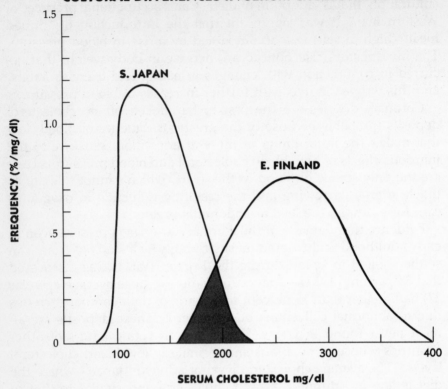

CULTURAL DIFFERENCES IN SERUM CHOLESTEROL LEVEL

Figure 1-3: Distribution frequency of serum cholesterol of men aged 40-59 in southern Japan and eastern Finland.

exceedingly high correlation existed between the average level of saturated fat consumed and the average cholesterol level within each country.

Data like these are among the best evidence of the preventability of coronary heart disease. Why do young and middle-aged Americans have heart disease, while in some other countries, the young and middle-aged do not? These differences cannot be attributed to ethnic factors; we know that migrating populations change their coronary risks to the extent that they acquire the health habits and risk factors of their adopted country. This has been shown for British, Norwegian, Irish, and Japanese immigrants in the United States, where all have developed higher heart attack rates than were present in their homelands.

The U.S. soldiers killed in Korea who had a 15 percent narrowing of coronary arteries were in no immediate danger of suffering premature coronary death. It takes another 15 to 30 years for atherosclerosis to take its toll. Fortunately, arteries can take a great deal of abuse. The vessels must close to a third of their original size (a 66 percent narrowing) before a clot (coronary thrombosis) can form that causes a true heart attack or that can lead to angina pectoris (chest pain upon effort, exposure to cold, or excitement).

The narrowing of Roger's arteries that began in his youth begins at an early age in the lives of millions of otherwise healthy people. Table 1-1 shows that after age 25, the number of deaths from heart disease and stroke increases in each age group until age 84 (after which the number drops because the pool of survivors is smaller).

Table 1-1: Number of Deaths from Heart Attacks and Strokes in the U.S. for Different Age Groups During 1983*

AGE DECADE	NUMBER OF DEATHS		
	Heart Attacks	*Strokes*	*Total*
25-34	1,000	1,000	2,000
35-44	7,000	2,000	9,000
45-54	26,000	5,000	31,000
55-64	75,000	13,000	88,000
65-74	139,000	30,000	169,000
75-84	172,000	55,000	227,000
Above 84	132,000	49,000	181,000
Total	552,000	155,000	707,000

*Figures to the nearest 1,000.

It is important to make clear that the goal of preventive medicine is not (and cannot be) to *extend* the normal life span—it is to allow us to *reach* it. People do have to die sometime. In *Vitality and Aging*, Drs. James Fries and Lawrence Crapo point out that average life expectancy will slowly move toward 85 from its present level of 75, with 95 percent of deaths occurring between ages 70 and 100. For many very elderly people heart attacks and strokes will likely be contributory causes of death.

Legendary pockets of healthy, active octogenarians attracted notice in a *National Geographic* article (January 1973) in which Dr. Alexander Leaf described three groups of long-lived peoples in mountainous regions of the Soviet Caucasus, the Himalayas, and the Ecuadorian Andes. These people tend to remain physically active throughout life and to eat foods consistently low in saturated fat and cholesterol. One problem with reports from these regions is that birth records are often nonexistent, and because those who can claim to have reached the age of 100 gain greatly increased social status, there is much suspicion that people add 10 or 20 years as they approach 80—and sometimes when they are much younger.

Even assuming that there is some truth to these reports of longevity, our goals in preventive medicine should be more modest. We should, however, be able to lower considerably our vulnerability to premature death and disability from heart disease. We have in fact already begun to reduce the impact of heart attacks and strokes by about 2 percent each year since the peak occurred in 1965. Lest we become too complacent, however, it is important to put this current downward trend into perspective. We still have a long way to go. If our national target is to reduce heart attack rates for the under-75 age group to one-tenth of our current rate (which is the current rate of Japan) that achievement—even at a 3 percent decline per year—would require 72 years. During this 72-year period, we would continue to acquiesce to the needless, premature death of almost 12 million individuals (a conservative figure based on the unlikely premise that the population does not increase during this period).

Through a concerted national effort, we can clearly accelerate the downward trend in heart disease. Sweden and Norway, for example, have embarked on national programs organized cooperatively by government, industry, and health groups, the goal of which is to eliminate smoking. Through another national program, Finland has already reduced the average intake of saturated fat. This was accomplished with the cooperation of the food industry in increasing production of lower-fat milk and cheese and production of lower-fat sausage.

The differing rate of death from heart disease among various countries and the fact that rates are likely to change suggest a second major reason why this epidemic is preventable: It is only since about 1900 that heart disease has emerged in industrialized nations of the world. Changing patterns of medical diagnosis confound certainty about the actual rate of increase of heart disease since 1900, but there is little doubt about the rarity of the problem before then. Although we in the United States have begun our decline, the heart disease epidemic has not yet peaked in countries that are still showing increases in various cardiovascular risk factors, such as smoking.

The Contribution of Smoking to Cardiovascular Risk

Roger's arteries received further abuse when he began his pack-a-day cigarette habit at age 23. When Roger began smoking, he was

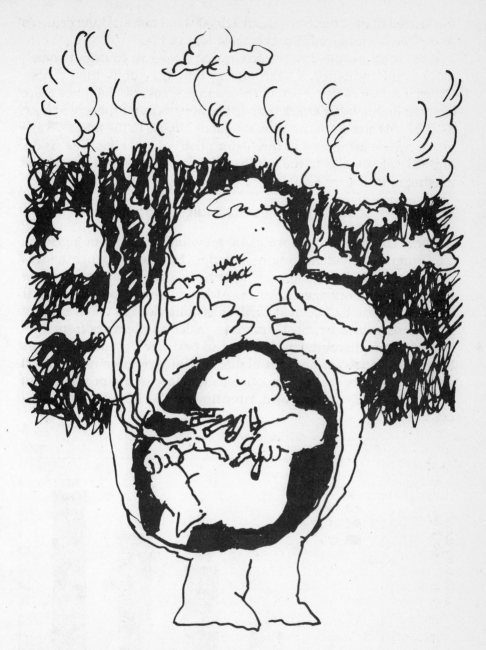

following the crowd; more than half of his peers had the habit. In the U.S. smoking by men of that age rose from about 20 percent in 1930 to a high of 66 percent in 1964. As we now know, this "normal" behavior contributes significantly to the incidence of lung cancer. In the United States, there are about 120,000 fatal cases of lung cancer a year. This is a tragic and preventable loss of life.

What most people don't realize is that cigarettes contribute much more to the incidence of heart attacks than they do to lung cancer. Other risk factors being equal, the average smoker is 2.4 times more likely to have a heart attack than is the nonsmoker. Probably at least 83,000 heart attacks of the annual total of 248,000 in the under-75 age group can be attributed to the "extra push" of smoking. The risk is impressively parallel to the number of cigarettes smoked per day, as illustrated in Figure 1-4.

Sedentary Living and Middle-Age Spread

Roger continued to smoke as he grew older, and in doing so he was progressively damaging his arteries. He married when he was 25 and followed the "normal" American pattern of gaining one pound a year from ages 25 to 48. At his death, he was 23 pounds heavier than he had been at 25. This is quite close to the average of 25 pounds gained by most American males and females from ages 20 to 50. It is discouraging that in the past few decades there has been a trend toward an even higher rate of weight gain among all American adults despite the obvious increase in the promotion of diet and exercise plans and attention to the health hazards of obesity.

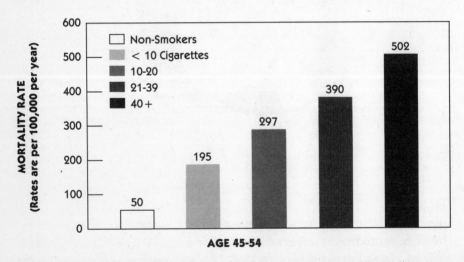

Figure 1-4: Coronary heart disease mortality rates by number of cigarettes currently smoked per day, men aged 45-54, U.S. veterans study, 1954-1962.

Because Roger shared the "normal" American tendency to become sedentary, some of his muscle mass had decreased and had been replaced by fat. Although Roger often watched sports, he seldom engaged in them. Consequently, his 23 pounds of weight gain probably constituted a gain of 30 pounds of fat, given perhaps seven pounds of muscle loss.

Roger's sedentary habits did more than allow his muscles to shrink; they allowed him to become needlessly overweight. Such habits are very likely the principal reason for obesity in the U.S. Dr. Henry Blackburn, one of the country's foremost cardiovascular epidemiologists, has pointed out that as a nation we are in fact consuming fewer calories than we did 50 to 75 years ago. Being overweight is, of course, due to consuming more calories than we burn, and the extraordinary decline in physical activity (largely a consequence of our love affair with the automobile) must be given the lion's share of the credit for our broad bottoms.

Daily Stress: Pressure to Do, Go, Succeed

Both as a child and as an adult, Roger was a hard-charging competitor. His family and teachers encouraged his achievement-oriented drives, and Roger rewarded them with a full measure of striving for grades, athletic honors, and professional advancement. He responded to pressure and stress by intensifying his efforts, and he accepted tension as an inevitable feature of his life. He did not capitulate to physical exhaustion or mental fatigue; he would press himself to his limits—and sometimes beyond. He frequently had more to do than time to do it in, and the stresses he bore became translated into flare-ups of outward anger or inward frustration.

Roger's career was a dynamic one, and the future promised even more. His family life was solid and a source of great satisfaction. Outwardly, he had everything going his way; he was both happy and successful. Still, despite the fact that Roger was rarely sick, his time-urgent, stressful life-style added daily to his preventable health burden. This, too, is typical of millions of people who, like Roger, lead highly pressured lives. The way daily stresses are managed is an important determinant of cardiovascular risk. Ineffective stress management can lead to elevated blood pressure levels and, to a lesser extent, elevated blood cholesterol.

At his checkup two years before his death, Roger's blood cholesterol and blood pressure levels were considered "normal," though in the upper range. He was further reassured by "normal" results of

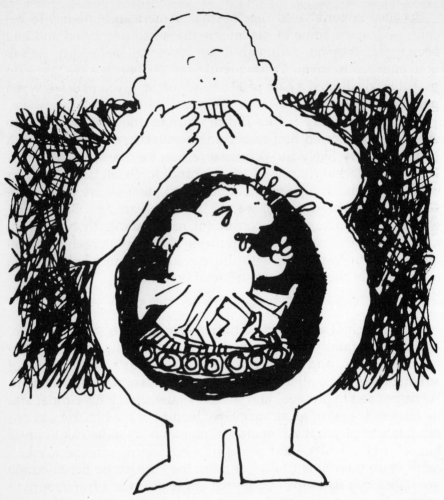

electrocardiograms taken when he was 45 and 46 years old. (Electrocardiograms, however, are not a very sensitive way to detect coronary artery narrowing.) Although Roger was given a clean bill of health, his one-pack-a-day cigarette habit and his high "normal" blood pressure and cholesterol levels, when considered together, increased his risk of heart attack to a level five times that of an individual whose risk factors are truly *normal*. The false attribution of normality to levels of cholesterol and blood pressure *because they are common in the U.S.* has led Dr. William Kannel of the Framingham Heart Project to say that "medical trivia kills." Risk factors clearly are additive, as is shown in Figure 1-5.

Case D is in fact Roger two years before his death. What is important for each individual to know is *how* risk factors get where they

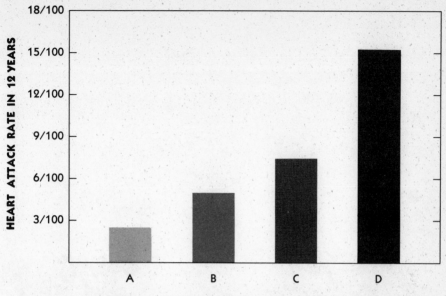

A = A nonsmoker, blood pressure 120/70 and cholesterol 170
B = Add one pack of cigarettes per day
C = Add high "normal" blood pressure, 140/88
D = Add high "normal" cholesterol, 250

Figure 1-5: The single and additive risk of heart attacks associated with smoking, cholesterol, and blood pressure in a 46-year-old man.

are and what can be done to lower them. But before we discuss how to reduce cardiovascular risk factors on both an individual and a family basis, it is important to identify the forces that push us in the wrong direction. Will they prevent us from quickening the current snail's pace of our decline in the epidemic of heart disease?

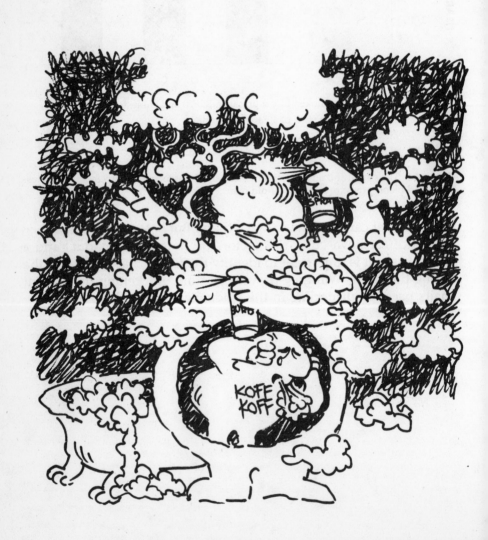

2

WHAT WENT WRONG?

During the past few decades, many aspects of the American dream have been challenged: our belief in growth as progress, our position as a world power, our confidence in our leaders and institutions, perhaps even our aspirations about ourselves and our potential. Despite this climate of scrutiny and reevaluation, one aspect of the American dream has survived intact—our basic confidence that the American way of life brings with it good health and the promise of a long life.

Epidemiologists—doctors concerned with the cause of the epidemic of stroke and heart disease—are painfully aware that the facts are quite different. Despite the undeniable and impressive decrease since 1900 in infant mortality and in infectious-disease mortality at all ages, there has been very little gain during this time in longevity for those who reach the age of 45. Since 1900, life expectancy from birth has increased about 20 years, whereas life expectancy for males who reach 45 has increased only about four years. Potential advances in life expectancy in the United States have been largely negated by the increase in premature cardiovascular deaths, though recent trends evidence a gradual lowering of such deaths. Unfortunately, lung cancer and the diet-related cancers (colon and breast) have not declined and continue to contribute to our burden of premature death and disability.

The heart disease epidemic has been sufficiently gradual to lull us into complacency about its presence. In his book *Man Adapting*, René Dubos points out that although our great capacity to adapt can be very beneficial, it can also lead us to tolerate and accept environmental changes that are deleterious to our well-being.

A case in point is provided by the notorious London fog. As Sherlock Holmes fans know, fog has been an indispensable part of London's character; mystery movies always include a suspenseful scene or two with unseen footsteps echoing through the fog. The thick, wet mist was not, however, a totally natural phenomenon. High concentrations of small particles distributed in the air bring about condensation of water vapor around them. This so-called fog was greatly compounded by and heavily laden with pollutants resulting from the burning of high-sulphur coal throughout London. For years British physicians treated something called "winter bronchitis" and were mystified that American physicians did not observe this illness in the United States. Why? The British had adapted to a man-made environmental problem. Although coal burning in London goes back to Roman times, it took modern growth of population and industrial pollution to create a setting in which a chronic situation could be identified. Eventually, a disaster occurred that jolted the British out of their complacency about the unhealthy air they breathed.

During the winter of 1952 a highly unusual temperature inversion resulted in a polluted fog of unprecedented thickness that lasted several days. Four thousand deaths over and above the statistical norm occurred in London, and the British awoke to the connection between the so-called fog and winter bronchitis as well as to the realization that they had long accepted a totally preventable scourge of pulmonary crippling. The problem was then given the priority it had long deserved, and it was solved: Winter bronchitis decreased markedly once the burning of high-sulphur coal was banned within the greater London area.

We seem to become immune to horrendous events when they are commonplace. From this perspective, it is instructive to project our statistics concerning premature death and disability from heart attacks and strokes onto a more dramatic screen. Let us say that beginning January 1, two jumbo jets crash every day of the year, killing 670 people per day (453 men, 217 women). The average age is 60, with an age range from 25 to 75. At the end of the year the total number of premature deaths from these airplane accidents is 248,000. In addition, another five jumbo jets crash daily, extensively injuring 1,643 people; after six months of intensive medical care, these crash victims are restored to only one-half of their pre-accident health and mobility. These non-fatal crashes involve a total of 600,000 persons by the end of the year. The total cost in lost earnings and medical care is about $100 billion. (The cost is increased by more than $2.0 billion if we subject 150,000 people to bone transplants that result in 7,000 operative deaths, 24,000 serious cripples, and more than 100,000 individuals who are partially disabled.)

The costs in the plane crash analogy are the actual estimated annual lost earnings and medical expenses of heart disease and stroke patients in the under-75 age group alone. The costs and complications of the fictitious transplants are analogous to the scope, costs, and results of the recent rapid development of surgery to bypass blocked coronary arteries. Such surgery is a modern technical solution to a problem that requires *prevention*, not just patchwork repair! Surgical repair is not a permanent solution to the damage of heart disease, and it does nothing for the 30 percent of all heart attack victims whose first heart attack is fatal.

Had such death and disability occurred because of airplane crashes, we as a nation would have restructured our priorities well before the year was out. We would have been horrified that such dreadful death and injury could occur and would have asked what could be done to prevent its recurrence. But because death and injury from heart disease have increased gradually since 1900, it is not readily apparent that we are experiencing an epidemic, or indeed that we have adapted to living patterns that bring with them totally unnecessary cardiovascular disease and death.

Compare this with the intense media attention given to any substance in the public food supply suspected of causing cancer. Quite justifiably, we become upset if we find we have been exposed to any unnecessary risk, even if no human lives are in fact lost. We expect the appropriate branches of the government to take action, and very often they do. And yet we stand by in silence while 679 Americans are killed each day, long before their time, by diseases known to be preventable!

AVOIDING UNPLEASANT REALITIES

Why are we not more alarmed by our chronic disease epidemic? Why have we adapted to the unacceptable?

We may to some extent be victims of our own success: While reductions in the rate of heart disease and stroke receive such good publicity, we tend to overlook the fact that the number of those affected is still unacceptably high. Part of the answer, too, is that people often suppress their awareness of unpleasant news. Many experiments have confirmed the fact that educational messages devised to arouse fear are counterproductive. People turn off their hearing and a mask of disinterest drops across their faces. Thoughts of getting cancer from smoking or of having a heart attack or stroke lend themselves to such suppression. The response can be instinctive: "It won't happen to me," or "Why think about it?" or "Everything is unhealthy these days," or "I've smoked too long to quit now." All of these reactions evade the basic realities. Individuals *can* take measures to live more healthily and with much greater energy and productivity. On an encouraging note, experiments have shown that counterproductive aspects of fear arousal decrease when warnings are coupled with specific instructions about how to solve a particular problem. Regrettably, many educational efforts to promote preventive medicine have been not only inadequate in scope but also faulty in their reliance on arousing fear; anti-smoking and seat-belt campaigns are instructive examples.

Deficient Nutritional Education

In identifying the causes of our adaptation to behavior patterns that are killing us, we find the classroom partly responsible. For decades, nutritional education in American schools has been based on a pervading fear of nutritional deficiencies—especially the lack of sufficient protein. As a result, a liberal intake of dairy foods, whole eggs, and meat has been promoted, leading to a "more is better" approach to nutrition. The California Dairy Association, an industry-supported group, has supplied extensive educational materials, for example, to state primary schools; the dollar value of those materials, if purchased by the public, has been estimated at $1 million per year. Similar programs exist in many other states. Although the quality of these educational materials is otherwise excellent, the messages exemplify the "avoid protein and calcium deficiency at all cost" type of teaching that has been the norm for years.

In the emphasis on protein consumption, there is usually no mention of potential harm—that the large amounts of whole milk, cheese, eggs, and meat that are recommended and the fats hidden in many foods such as pastry might introduce saturated-fat and cholesterol intakes that contribute to atherosclerosis. Nor is it usually mentioned that making intelligent choices among those foods can avert potential damage. Most Americans do not know, for example, that most of the protein in an egg is in the white and that all the cholesterol is in the yolk. They often do not know that the vegetable shortening on the label of many prepared foods is often a hydrogenated fat, which means that it is saturated and will raise blood cholesterol levels. These simple distinctions should be part of everyone's nutritional education—as should be the fact that other sources of protein such as fish, poultry, lean meats, or legumes (beans, peas, lentils) offer alternative ways to keep saturated-fat intake at desirable levels. The role of excessive sugar and salt in contributing to cardiovascular disease is another vital subject that has been largely ignored in nutritional education in our elementary, secondary, and high schools.

Eating Habits Acquired in Childhood

Another potential source of bad eating habits goes back even further than grade school. It involves the foods you grew up eating, liking, and wanting as a child and the eating habits you acquired. Did you have to clean your plate? Were your foods highly salted or sugared? Did you eat lots of red meat and dairy products every day? Were soft drinks, cookies, and other sweets readily available? Food preferences are established early. If you were raised on a diet high in sugar, salt and saturated fat, you probably enjoy such food. Unfortunately, this kind of diet starts you on a path to coronary heart disease. With proper knowledge and specific skills, however, people can change not only harmful eating habits but also the foods they enjoy eating.

The Influence of Advertising

The foods you grew up eating and liking provide a mini-reflection of American food preferences and eating habits. Visitors to the United States are often overwhelmed by certain vivid first impressions of our culture. They frequently comment on the ingenuity, persuasiveness, and pervasiveness of advertising devoted to food. Such advertising has a powerful influence on eating habits—especially those of children. The average child sees more than 20,000 commercials a year, of which as many as 13,000 are for food or beverages.

The food industry's advertising budget for 1985 has been estimated at about $5 billion. Money available from other sources to promote an objective view of good nutrition through the mass media is almost nonexistent. Since nutritional education in schools is often inadequate, the influence of food advertising on shaping our eating habits should not be underestimated.

The bulk of food advertising is devoted to pushing highly processed convenience foods, which are often heavily sugared or salted and often have saturated fats added to them. A large amount of fat, most often saturated, is also present in many baked products. Most people are not aware of these *hidden fats* and often believe that they are consuming a high carbohydrate food without realizing that a large percentage of the calories frequently comes from fats. Nutritionist Dr. Jean Mayer, president of Tufts University, pointed out in *U.S. Nutrition Policies in the Seventies* that these heavily sugared, salted, and otherwise modified foods comprised over 55 percent of our total intake (compared to 10 percent in 1941). Mayer believes that this increased consumption is largely a result of advertising. Although other factors cannot be overlooked (time saved in food preparation, etc.), advertising not only brings about shifts between brands but may well promote shifts in our eating styles.

Recent phenomena that are an increasingly important determinant of our food-consumption patterns are the decisions on food choices made by fast-food chains. If advertising has a role in determining consumer preferences, then the budget increase in advertising expenditures from $5 million in 1967 to $450 million in 1984 for McDonald's restaurant chain exemplifies a powerful commercial force. Hamburger and french fries consumption in the United States has risen sharply in the past 20 years, and fast-food chains are a significant factor in this increase. McDonald's alone now serves 6 percent of the population of the United States *every day*!

The Tobacco Industry

Another factor linked to the acquiring of bad health habits is the tobacco industry. There are approximately 51 million citizens in the United States who smoke cigarettes (including 19 percent of high school seniors). Three-quarters of all smokers say they want to quit, and in the past year 37 percent of current smokers actually attempted to quit. Another 15 percent of smokers say they would try to quit if easier ways of doing so were available. However, resources allocated to the promotion of smoking continue to far outweigh those spent to discourage it. The United States Public Health Service has raised its spending on smoking control from $2.2 million in 1976 to $37.9 million in 1985, but this is no match for the promotion and advertising budget of the tobacco industry, which reached $2.65 billion in 1983. Ever alert to new markets, the industry has targeted young women to "come a long way" to the devastation caused by cigarette smoking. The rise of 95 percent since 1969 in sales of smokeless tobacco (snuff and chewing tobacco) reflects new users in the 15-25 age group. This new market will lead to addiction to nicotine and to many new cases of cancer of the mouth. Our young people are lured into using these products by means of innovative advertising methods that involve sporting events, sports figures, and celebrities in the entertainment industry. Meanwhile, the American tobacco industry still benefits from federal subsidies to the tune of $100 million in 1983. Where will the muscle and dollars come from to counteract the power and influence of the American tobacco industry?

Tobacco was the first important cash crop of the United States. In 1984, the sale of tobacco products by the top five U.S. tobacco companies amounted to $25 billion, yielding pre-tax profits of approximately $4.6 billion (and after-tax profits of roughly $2.8 billion). It is a matter of public record that politicians from tobacco-producing states have consistently opposed legislation that would impair the growth and lower federal support for the tobacco industry.

Automation

Another aspect of our modern American life-style may have contributed to a more vigorous economy but to weaker, flabbier bodies. The growing urbanization and mechanization of modern life have made it easier for us to become physically lazy and sedentary. We drive rather than walk; we take an elevator rather than climb stairs; we push a button on an electric dryer rather than bend down and reach up to hang clothes on a clothesline. The average American takes a car for any trip more than two blocks long! Whereas exercise was once an inevitable part of living, today we must consciously plan to get the exercise needed to maintain good health.

Over the past 50 years, though our calorie intake has actually fallen, the prevalence of overweight has risen, largely owing to our more sedentary habits. Increased physical activity can provide an important remedy. The one to two pounds of weight gained yearly from ages 20 to 50 by the average adult can be prevented by as little as ten extra minutes of brisk walking per day.

Scientific Conservatism

Scientific conservatism is another influence that can contribute to our passive adaptation to preventable cardiovascular death and disability. This conservatism is two-pronged. First, there is an inevitable time lag between a discovery and the synthesis of that discovery into coherent action. For example, sufficient evidence to implicate cigarettes in lung cancer and heart attacks existed for at least five years before the Surgeon General's 1964 report that officially proclaimed cigarettes a health hazard. The most effective counter to this time lag is education, inside and outside the scientific establishment.

Second, an underlying conviction held by a large proportion of medical researchers is that all the pieces of the puzzle should be at hand before making the first move to devise coherent action. The most effective counter to this "let's wait for complete proof" attitude is exemplified by the comment of the late Donald Reid of the London School of Hygiene and Tropical Medicine: "Don't let the best be the enemy of the good." Although it is desirable to know *why* cigarettes cause cancer, this goal should not become the enemy of devising ways to help prevent people from starting to smoke as well as ways to help current smokers kick their habit.

Research should of course continue to try to identify the ingredients of cigarette smoke that cause cancer, the characteristics that influence susceptibility to the disease, and the cellular mechanisms of cancer formation. These kinds of basic research advance our knowledge and might, for example, lead to benefits relevant to the prevention of treatment of other kinds of cancer.

Thus, we should continue to support basic research while *simultaneously* implementing our best efforts for appropriate preventive measures, rather than sit passively and wait for basic research to yield conclusive findings on *all* facets of the complex puzzle.

The combination of a normal lag and a "let's wait" attitude can erect impressive barriers to preventive action. Barry Commoner, in his book, *The Closing Circle*, speaks of the need for closing the circle of ecological reality. By this he means that the final cost of industrial growth must include the cost to the consumer of repairing the damage or recycling the waste materials of the products consumed. Closing the circle in medical care requires efforts geared to prevention, accompanied by the necessary educational and political supports. We currently expend much more money and effort learning about the causes of diseases and methods of repairing their damage than on ways of preventing people from getting the diseases in the first place.

We clearly need more resources allocated to preventive medicine. These resources will come only via the public's demand transmitted through political action. As Professor Victor Fuchs of Stanford points out in his book *Who Shall Live?* an economist's view of problems of resource allocation is tempered by the realism that resources are finite. What is needed, therefore, is an appraisal of the current allocation of resources to various facets of medical research, followed by action to close the glaring gap between research on the causes of disease and the preventive action needed to support better public health. The following chart depicts the sequence of events needed to close the circle of public health (from problem identification to problem solution).

SEQUENCE FOR SOLUTION OF A PUBLIC HEALTH PROBLEM

Problem Identification — — — — — —▶ Problem Solution
▼
Basic Research on Cause
▼
Field Research on Treatment
or Prevention
▼
Education of Public and Health
Professionals on Treatment
or Prevention
▼
Legislative or Voluntary
Changes in Society

There is an apocryphal story about a man preoccupied with rescuing drowning victims from a river who, when asked what was happening, replied in exhaustion, "I don't know; I've been too busy to find out who's been pushing them in upstream." We currently have a partial repair system in our burgeoning medical establishment that is predominantly "downstream." Despite the excellence of our medical care system, and despite the fact that the growth rate of our medical care costs for the past decade has been twice that of our Gross National Product, there is a growing consensus that closing the circle will require a decision to channel resources to primary prevention.

Recently there has been a decided swing toward this point of view as evidenced by many local and state initiatives, health promotion programs in worksites, and impressive government documents, such as the 1979 publications of *Healthy People: The Surgeon General's*

Report on Health Promotion and Disease Prevention, followed in 1984 by *Prospects for a Healthier America*, published by the U.S. Department of Health and Human Services. An excellent summary of these expanded federal government activities appears in *Prevention '84/85*, published by the Office of Disease Prevention and Health Promotion of the U.S. Public Health Service, an effective organization of the government, ably led by Dr. J. Michael McGinnis. The National Institutes of Health has convened many national conferences—known as *consensus conferences*. These led to the publication of important reports on current opinions on major disease-prevention issues such as osteoporosis, obesity, and cholesterol and heart disease.

However, we still don't have our national priorities right. As pointed out by Dr. Alvin Tarlov of the Kaiser Family Foundation, only 0.3 percent of our total health care costs of $460 billion per year are spent on preventive services, despite the fact that 67 percent of all disease is preventable.

Will Rogers once said we would be the only nation in history to go to the poorhouse in an automobile. To that I might add, we are the only nation in the world to go to the bank in an ambulance. Despite our colossal Gross National Product, our average wage earner's income in 1984 of $15,720 per year, our magnificent hospitals, our abundant corn and wheat belts, and our trips to the moon, today's middle-aged adult can expect to live only about four years longer than did his or her counterpart in 1900. Furthermore, needless suffering from chronic illness has increased over this time period. The dream of abundant good health and satisfying quality of life has remained outside our reach. It need not. It is merely a matter of national choices and priorities—and of each of us taking the initiative to adopt a healthy life-style.

REVERSIBILITY OF ATHEROSCLEROSIS

As encouragement for embarking on a program to lower cardiovascular risk factors, it is important to know that the atherosclerotic process that slowly chokes off arteries (and life) is not only preventable but also, to an important degree, *reversible* both in humans and in certain closely related species.

Evidence from Animal Experiments

Drs. Marc Armstrong, Emory Warner, and William Connor of the Universities of Iowa and Oregon have conducted careful and con-

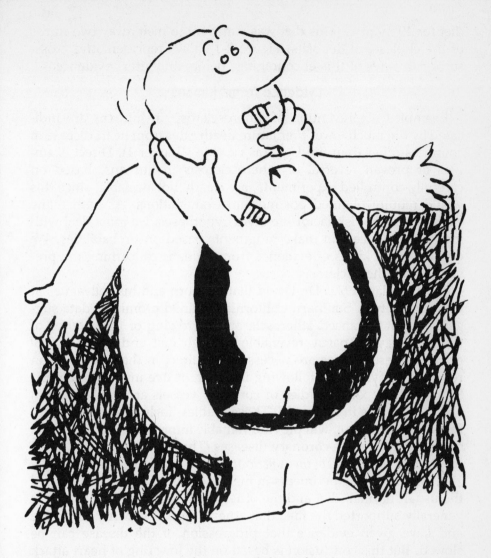

vincing experiments on the reversibility of artherosclerosis in animals. In studies undertaken from 1963 to 1969 they found an average
narrowing of 60 percent in the main coronary arteries of 20 adult
rhesus monkeys after 17 months of feeding them diets high in
saturated fat and cholesterol. These diets raised the animals' blood
cholesterol levels from the normal monkey cholesterol level of 140 to
about 705.

The most remarkable findings concerned the effects of diet on
reversibility. After 17 months on the atherosclerosis-producing
(atherogenic) diet, another 20 monkeys were switched to a normal

diet for 40 months. This diet was sufficient to melt away two-thirds of the cholesterol deposits. Figure 2-1 shows representative cross-sectional views of this encouraging "before-and-after" evidence.

Evidence from Humans

Examples of prevention of atherosclerosis in humans are indicated by the much lower premature death rates from heart disease in countries other than the U.S. (as cited in Chapter 1). Direct examples of proven reversal of atherosclerosis in humans, based on carefully controlled experiments, are clearly not available, since this would require planned postmortem examinations. As with many elements of the risk-factor/life-style hypotheses, we must deal with indirect evidence and make judgments based on probabilities. We do have three kinds of evidence from humans concerning the prevention of atherosclerosis:

1. In the late 1970s Dr. David Blankenhorn and his colleagues at the University of Southern California obtained promising data suggesting that advanced atherosclerotic narrowing of the arteries of the legs may be partly reversible through diet and exercise programs. (These studies are necessarily indirect in that they rely on repeated x-ray studies following injection of dye into the arteries.) Similar repeat x-ray studies of coronary vessels are in progress in about 15 centers in the world. These studies, including one at Stanford Medical School, will provide valuable information on the effects of diet and drugs on coronary diseases. The first results were documented in *The Journal of the American Medical Association* in June 1987.

2. More direct experiments in matched groups of adults—one fed the usual "normal" diet and the other a low-saturated-fat diet—have generally supported the idea that atherosclerosis is partly reversible and have given evidence that progression of the disease can be slowed. But this conclusion is based on the lowering of heart attack rate only. Similar studies on the influence of diet or drugs have been done in Norway, Belgium, the United States, and Finland. All are consistent with the hypothesis that lowering of cardiovascular risk factors decreases the incidence of heart disease.

3. Unplanned experiments or opportunities provided by nature have added to the consistency and congruence of the cardiovascular risk-factor argument. These experiments consist of data from occupied Norway and Holland and from Great Britain during World War II that showed transient but surprisingly prompt reduction in deaths attributed to cardiovascular disease beginning a few years

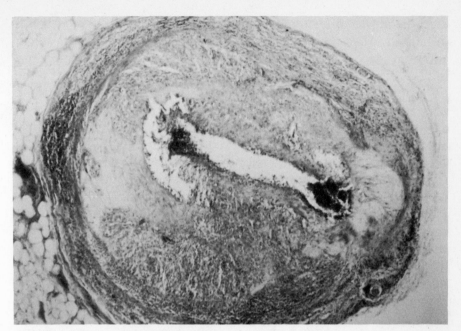
After 17 months on a high-cholesterol diet.

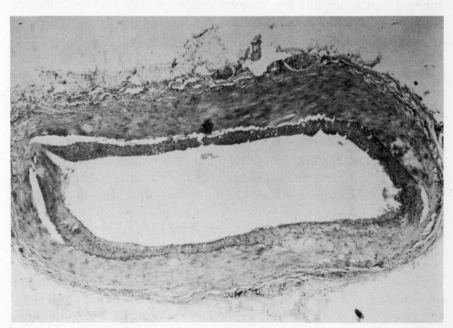
After 17 months on a high-cholesterol diet, followed by 40 months on a normal monkey diet.

Figure 2-1: Arteries of cholesterol-fed monkeys.

after the abrupt life-style changes associated with the war were set in motion. These changes included reduced intake of meat, sugar, and dairy products, as well as decreased cigarette consumption and increased physical activity. Additional evidence is provided by the prompt rise in heart attack deaths that occurred in postwar Europe several years after the return to the prewar relative abundance of cigarettes, meat, sugar, and dairy products and the reduced physical activity due to greater use of automobiles.

In the United States, it is encouraging to note that voluntary life-style changes have contributed to the significant decrease in the occurrence of heart attacks and strokes since 1965. Millions of people *are* exercising more, keeping their weight down, eating a low-saturated-fat diet, and giving up smoking.

Doctors, for example, have dramatically changed their smoking habits since the publication of the Surgeon General's report in 1964. According to a survey conducted in 1973 by the journal *Medical Economics*, about two-thirds of previously smoking physicians had stopped. Even greater changes have occurred since then. It is now rare to see doctors smoking at national meetings, whereas the smoke-filled room of 25 years ago testified to the fact that doctors were representative of the national smoking average — 55 percent of adult men and about 15 percent of adult women smoked at that time.

In the population at large, the percentage of smokers over the age of 20 has decreased from 42.7 percent in 1965 to 32 percent in 1983. Unfortunately, there was a sharp increase in the number of women smokers in that period, from about 15 percent to 29 percent. Indeed, female high-school students are now more likely to smoke than males (with 20.5 percent of the girls reporting that they smoke compared with 16 percent of the boys). Smoking rates for adult women, however, like those for men, are now showing a sharp decline.

Although complete data are not available, casual inspection tells us that many adult Americans have acquired a habit that is beneficial to the lowering of at least two of the three major risk factors — a habit of regular, sustained physical activity of the sort that increases cardiovascular fitness and lowers body weight and blood cholesterol (and is usually accompanied by the cessation of cigarette smoking). This type of exercise is exemplified by the joggers and bicyclists who have now become a familiar part of the American landscape. In the United States there are now more bicycles sold each year than passenger cars, and according to the Bicycle Manufacturers Association of America there are more than four times as many cyclists in this country as there were in 1960 — a trend that further attests to the growing number of Americans young and old who are exercising more.

Other changes have occurred in dietary habits of the American public during the past 15 years, owing to the increased nationwide interest in nutrition and obesity control. These include a shift from butter to margarine and from whole milk to low-fat and nonfat milk, a drop in egg consumption, and a decreased intake of beef, though cheese consumption has risen considerably. The net effect of these dietary changes is the probable cause of a modest reduction in the cholesterol levels of adults during the past 15 years. The rising interest in weight control is demonstrated by the growth of weight-control organizations. The nonprofit self-help group TOPS (Take Off Pounds Sensibly) has acquired 308,000 members since its inception 40 years ago. Equally impressive is the rise in membership in Weight Watchers, which now numbers over 650,000.

We should be challenged by our own success and by the experiences of other countries. It is apparent that *the American way of life need not be hazardous to your health*. It is time for the citizen-consumer to become informed sufficiently to take personal responsibility for maintaining his or her own health.

But if we have at our disposal the *information* to accomplish this, can we also acquire the *skills* to lower chronic disease risk at an individual and a family level? Yes. This book is designed to help you achieve your personal goals to live a healthier and more productive life and to avoid the needless risk of many chronic diseases, including heart attack, stroke, osteoporosis, diabetes, and many forms of cancer.

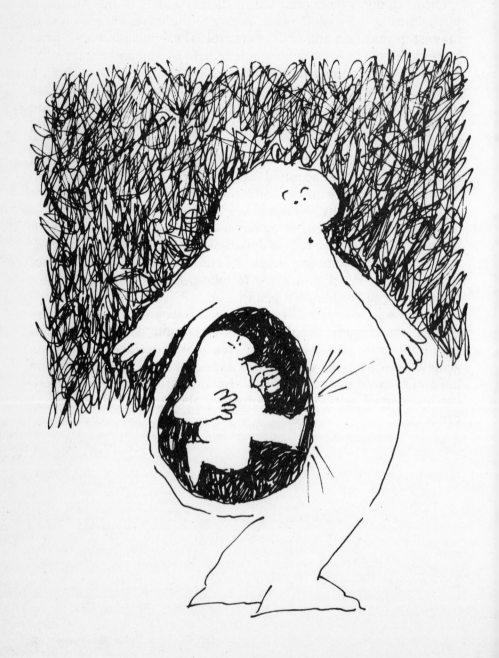

3

ACHIEVING
SELF-DIRECTED CHANGE

T he individual or family that wishes to change long-estab-
lished health habits can learn the skills of behavior change.
The methods are surprisingly simple and rewarding. This
chapter introduces these skills and the principles on which
they are based; they will be discussed in more detail in subsequent
chapters as they apply to the lowering of specific risk factors.

It seems to be human nature to want something for nothing. Yet
though basic health maintenance in our culture is free, we insist on
paying. The cost to repair the damage from largely preventable
ailments cannot be measured in mere financial terms. The needless
human suffering is staggering. We buy diet foods, follow crash
diets, swallow diet pills; we undergo expensive operations (such as
a coronary bypass) to repair something that need not have been
damaged in the first place. We rely on chemicals to calm us during
the day and to help us sleep at night, without trying to change the
sources of our stress. We learn to depend upon external cures—
healers, pills, machines—rather than to rely more upon ourselves to
practice preventive medicine.

For decades, many family doctors have sincerely tried to help
patients lose weight, lower blood pressure, reduce stress, and
change dietary and activity habits adverse to good health. They have
felt pleased and satisfied when a patient has responded to their
professional advice and have been disappointed and often saddened
when sickness or death have been the victors.

The physician brings to his patients the fullness of his knowledge
and professional experience. He carries his years of training with

him. When he treats a patient, he acts on the faith that he is doing the best he can. Yet somewhere in the relationship between the patient and the physician, between the patient and the entire health-care system, between good health and poor health, lies a weak link. The weak link is not the disease, not the medicine, not the surgery, not all the decisions by the physician; it is that critical and often disregarded task of the individual to take responsibility for maintaining his or her own health. This is not an overwhelming task. One of the great benefits of modern behavioral research has been the development of skills and techniques the individual can acquire to help himself.

We need to stop making excuses and we need to stop expecting a cure-all somewhere "out there" to compensate for unhealthy living patterns. The daily life-style choices that we make are shaped by a powerful complex of influences within our culture. The forces in our popular culture that promote, create, and maintain ill health are obvious when they appear in advertising to promote smoking; they are not so obvious when they appear at a second level of influence – for example, the chance association of children with a smoking peer group (the single most important determinant of smoking adoption by teenagers).

Because our environment does surround us with deleterious influences, we need skills to use in self-defense. Within the last few years, we have gathered confirming evidence that skills needed for life-style changes can be systematically and readily taught and learned and that the individual need not depend upon that mystical and unmeasurable factor called willpower to change deep-rooted habits. It is actually better for our emotions and more productive for our health to forget about willpower, with its Calvinistic connotations, and embrace instead the skills of behavior modification. I prefer to call the process "achieving self-directed change" – the phrase suggested by behavioral psychologist Albert Bandura of Stanford University – because the individual makes the changes while the book or educator supplies the concepts to be learned and practiced.

In some circles, the mere mention of behavior modification evokes visions of Orwell's 1984, complete with Big Brother, thought control, and loss of personal freedom. But such a vision is a woeful misinterpretation. In fact, the principles and learning skills acquired to achieve self-directed change are liberating influences that can wrest an individual from habits that enslave him. When the current healthy minority of our population (nonsmokers, healthy eaters, exercisers, effective stress managers) becomes the majority, the popular culture will naturally reinforce health—and the benefits of good living, including good health, will be easier to achieve.

METHODS FOR ACHIEVING SELF-DIRECTED CHANGE

When embarking on a program to lower chronic disease risk factors, carry out in sequence the steps that follow and repeat them as often as needed. Before you begin, it is important, however, that you adopt the attitude that a change would be worth the required effort. You will then be ready to proceed along a six-stage program: (1) identifying the problem; (2) building confidence and commitment to change; (3) increasing your awareness of behavior patterns by self-observation; (4) developing and implementing an action plan; (5) evaluating your plan; and (6) maintaining the changes you have brought about. This sequence was developed by behavioral psychologist Carl Thoresen of Stanford.

ONE: IDENTIFYING THE PROBLEM

Self-directed change first requires that you identify the nature of the problem. Begin this process by taking the simplified self-scoring test on pages 38-39 which enables you to gain insight into your chronic disease risk factors and the health habits that underlie them. The risk factor of high blood cholesterol, for instance, is linked to a cluster of causes: lack of exercise, excess dietary saturated fat and cholesterol, caloric excess and sedentary habits (leading to obesity or overweight), and, to a lesser extent, stressful living, high sugar intake, and low fiber intake. The risk factor of elevated blood pressure is linked to excess salt in the food, stressful living, and the poor exercise and eating habits that contribute to overweight.

Your priorities for choices of health habits to observe will flow naturally from an effective and reasonably accurate method of gauging your areas of highest chronic disease risk. This may require a period of self-observation. Smokers, for instance, may need to record the number of packs they purchase over a period of a few weeks (though most confirmed smokers, when questioned, know within 20 percent what their actual intake is). To assess accurately salt, sugar, saturated-fat, and cholesterol intakes, a knowledge of food composition and a period of self-observation are necessary. But at this beginning stage, make a preliminary assessment of your chronic

SIMPLIFIED SELF-SCORING TEST OF CHRONIC DISEASE RISK

Risk habit or factor	Increasing risk				
1. Smoking Cigarettes	None	Up to 9 per day	10 to 24 per day	25 to 34 per day	35 or more per day
Score	0	1	2	3	4
2. Body Weight	Ideal Weight	Up to 9 lbs. excess	10 to 19 lbs. excess	20 to 29 lbs. excess	30 lbs. or more excess
Score	0	1	2	3	4
3. Salt Intake	1/5 average	1/3 average	U.S. average	Above average	Far above average
or	hard to achieve; no added salt; no convenience foods	no use of salt at table, spare use of high-salt foods	salt in cooking, some salt at table	frequent salt at table	frequent use of salty foods
Blood Pressure Upper Reading (if known)	Less than 110	110 to 129	130 to 139	140 to 149	150 or over
Score	0	1	2	3	4
4. Saturated Fat and Cholesterol Intake	1/5 average	1/3 average	1/2 average	U.S. average	Above average
or	almost total vegetarian; rare egg yolk, butterfat and lean meat	2 meatless days/week, no whole milk products, lean meat only	meat (mostly lean), eggs, cheese 12 times/week, nonfat milk only	meat, cheese, eggs, whole milk 24 times/ week	meat, cheese, eggs, whole milk over 24 times/week
Blood Cholesterol Level (if known)	Less than 150	150 to 169	170 to 199	200 to 219	220 or over
Score	0	1	2	3	4

disease risk level. The results of this test will allow you to set your initial goals.

More complete and more accurate scoring systems will appear in subsequent chapters and will be useful in later stages of your program. In the simplified self-scoring test, the six primary risk factors involved in cardiovascular and other chronic diseases are listed and a score of 0 to 4 is given for each (with a theoretical maximum of 24 points possible). Do not skip this test. Take it in an experimental spirit, since neither your initial self-observation nor the relative risk is precise. This score does, however, effectively set the stage for more careful self-observation, which will allow a more accurate self-appraisal and hence a more accurate score.

Risk habit or factor			Increasing risk		
5. Self-rating of Physical Activity or Walking Rating	Vigorous exercise 4 or more times/week 20 min. each Brisk walking 5 times/week 45 min. each	Vigorous exercise 3 times/week 20 min. each Brisk walking 3 times/week 30 min. each	Vigorous exercise 1 to 2 times/week Brisk walking 2 times/week 30 min. each or Normal walking 4-1/2 to 6 miles daily	U.S. average occasional exercise Normal walking 2-1/2 to 4-1/2 miles daily	Below average exercises rarely Normal walking less than 2-1/2 miles daily
Score	0	1	2	3	4
6. Self-rating of Stress and Tension	Rarely tense or anxious or Yoga, meditation, or equivalent 20 min. 2 times/day	Calmer than average Feel tense about 3 times/ week	U.S. average Feel tense or anxious 2 to 3 times/day Frequent anger or hurried feelings	Quite tense Usually rushed Occasionally take tranquilizer	Extremely tense Take tranquilizer 5 times/week or more
Score	0	1	2	3	4

Enter your total score here _____ .

Notes: 1) Subtract 1 point if dietary fiber intake is high (almost all cereals whole grain, almost no sugar, and considerable fruit and vegetable intake). 2) If you are a female taking estrogen or birth control pills, add 1 point if score is 12 or below, 2 points if risk score is 13 or above (especially if you smoke, are overweight, have high blood pressure or high blood cholesterol). 3) Add 1 point for each 10 points of blood pressure above 150 and 1 point for each 30 points of cholesterol above 220. 4). Subtract 1 point if high density cholesterol level (the protective cholesterol fraction that increases with exercise) is greater than 50.

In calculating ideal weight in this test, I suggest formulae adapted from those recommended by Michael and Kathryn Mahoney in their book *Permanent Weight Control*: for women, ideal weight = height in inches × 3.5 – 108; for men, ideal weight = height in inches × 4 – 128. Thus, the ideal weight for a woman who is 5′5″ is 119½ pounds. (This method is useful for people of average build. People who are either stocky or slight in build will find it helpful to look at alternative ways to assess their excess weight, as described in Chapter 7.)

For categories 3 and 4 of the test, your self-rating (your habitual salt intake or estimated fat intake) is preferable to actual measurements (blood pressure or blood cholesterol). Focusing on the habit (behavior) is more relevant to our task because measurements, such as blood pressure and blood cholesterol, are the dual result of the behavior patterns *and* of genetic factors over which one has no control. A further problem with reliance on blood pressure or blood cholesterol values is their variability (from day to day for cholesterol and even from minute to minute for blood pressure). Hence, when using such measurements it is desirable to average at least three measurements. Unfortunately, most people rarely have such data available. Another problem with blood pressure and blood cholesterol data is that they are quite often inaccurate, due to errors in measurement that are usually not evident to the measurer. Because of these limitations, you may wish to assess yourself using both methods (self-rating and actual measurement) and average the two.

Studies undertaken in the Stanford Center for Research in Disease Prevention and elsewhere have indicated that women who take estrogen pills or birth control pills incur increased cardiovascular risk related to the metabolic effects that estrogen has on the body. Both estrogen pills and birth control pills tend to elevate blood pressure and plasma cholesterol levels. Estrogen increases salt retention, which in turn increases blood pressure. And although natural progesterone has diuretic properties, synthetic progesterone (used in birth control pills along with estrogen) increases salt retention. Cardiovascular risks associated with estrogen and birth control pill use are additive: Women who already have high blood cholesterol, high blood pressure, who smoke or are overweight face many times the cardiovascular risk of thin, nonsmoking women with normal blood pressure and blood cholesterol levels.

INTERPRETATION

(Risks are given for cardiovascular disease. They apply, but with less precision, for adult-onset diabetes and diet-related cancers of the breast and colon. For smoking-related cancer of the lungs, the predominant risk is duration and amount of smoking.)

Zone	Score	(Maximum points = 24)
F	20-24	The probability of having a premature heart attack or stroke is about four to five times the U.S. average. Action is urgent. Try to drop four points within a month and three more points within six months.

E	16-19	Incidence of heart attack or stroke is about twice the U.S. average. Action is urgent. Try to drop four points within six months and continue reduction.
D	12-15	The U.S. average is 13. This is an uncomfortable and readily avoidable zone. Careful planning can result in a five- to six-point reduction within a year.
C	8-11	The likelihood of having a heart attack or stroke is about one-half the U.S. average. This is a zone rather easily achieved by most people within a year if they are now in zone D or E. Careful planning can result in a four- to six-point reduction within a year.
B	4-7	Incidence of heart attack or stroke about one-quarter of the U.S. average. This goal is achievable by many but often takes one or two years to reach.
A	0-3	Incidence of heart attack or stroke rates very low, averaging less than one-tenth the rate in the U.S. 35–65 age group. This goal requires diligent effort, considerable family support, and often takes three to four years to reach. Individuals in this range should be proud and gratified (and will often find themselves acting as models and teachers for the many who have not achieved this very low-risk zone).

After completing the self-scoring test most people will find ample room for health habit changes in at least four of the six risk habits or risk factors. The remainder of this chapter takes you through the rest of a prototype risk-reduction procedure, borrowing from examples you will find more fully described in later chapters. Suppose that you recognize that a problem exists, for example, after noting that your level of physical activity is exceedingly low (a pedometer reading averaging less than two and one-half miles per day after a week of observation). Let us also suppose that you are 15 pounds overweight and that you wish to control your weight by increasing your level of physical activity and lowering your caloric intake.

At this stage it would be useful to make a formal, conscious decision to act and to consider specific ways to give this decision extra commitment. Recognize, for instance, that it is easy to over-estimate good intentions. Do not assume your commitment is strong enough; instead, try to formulate ways to strengthen it. Writing a "self-contract," which reinforces your decision and which (if possible) enlists the aid of a helper, is one important way to build commitment. Realize that some highly structured step, even one that feels "artificial," may be crucial to get yourself moving. Try not to be bothered by the formal connotations of a "contract"; think of it as a list of plans. A self-contract may be quite brief and to the point — simply that you are going to plan a program. In general, self-contracts should be designed for intervals of a week or two, because short-term goals are more readily attained. Feel free to revise your contract after a few days if your experience suggests changes are needed.

After making your initial commitment to attempt a change, you are ready for the next stage of problem identification: analyzing your potential barriers to change. Despite an awakening of concern about and interest in changing various habits, you may be rather content with your old habits — for example, a sedentary life-style. You may be subconsciously proud to reflect the view that Robert Hutchins once expressed: "Whenever I get the urge to exercise, I sit down until it goes away." You may move (or not move) in circles of similarly sedentary friends and may even think people will regard you as some sort of faddist or health freak if you embark on an exercise program, especially one using written contracts and other structured methods.

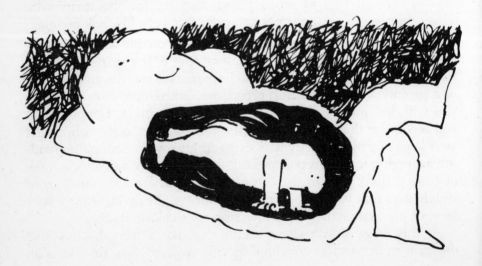

These are "belief barriers" that need to be overcome. Your prior belief may well have been, "That's just the way I am." But both attitudes and behavior are changeable—though not without sustained attention and effort. Modern behavioral science has demonstrated that you *can* change deleterious attitudes and behaviors through conscious and systematic application of specific techniques. These techniques allow you to change how you think, how you talk to yourself, how you react, and how you use "self-instructions."

Gaining better control of one's own mind is a goal that has fascinated man for centuries, but for years many behavioral scientists remained aloof from anything that could not be readily observed and recorded. The recent advances in behavioral science that have led to better understanding of self-control have come from psychologists who have pioneered methods for training our own thinking practices—our internal mental environment. Among those pioneers are behavioral psychologists Michael Mahoney of Pennsylvania State University and Carl Thoresen. Although many people realize that they frequently daydream or talk to themselves, few know how influential these internal monologues are in controlling their everyday adjustments to life.

In *Permanent Weight Control* the Mahoneys identify and label many common mental pitfalls that afflict overweight individuals. They describe the very common problem caused by perfectionist goal setting, which leads to discouragement ("I blew it") and hence to negative or maladaptive monologues ("I'm no good"), and from there to binge eating or snacking with a vengeance.

You can modify your internal monologues to reinforce behavior change by learning a set of thinking skills useful in coping with stress—breaking a smoking habit, launching and maintaining an exercise program, changing your food patterns, and achieving weight control. (Specific examples of such self-monologues are given in later chapters.)

All phases of the self-directed change process will draw on this ability to modify your own internal monologues or self-instructions. Why? Because this will enable you to identify problems more accurately, build commitment, and become more aware of your experiences. The chart on page 44 provides examples of rather common negative self-monologues that act as barriers to potential changes; alternative positive statements follow.

You may want to devote a few days to ferreting out your attitudes about the feasibility of changing some of your behavior patterns.

THOUGHTS THAT IMPEDE OR PROMOTE
A WILLINGNESS TO BEGIN CHANGE

Risk Factor Area		Examples of Positive and Negative Self-Talk
Exercise	Negative:	I don't have the time to exercise. I'm afraid I'd look silly.
	Positive:	A walk around the block before dinner would be relaxing.
Smoking	Negative:	I'm afraid I'd gain weight if I stopped smoking. I've smoked too long to give it up now.
	Positive:	I can learn new techniques to quit smoking that have been effective in helping other people break the habit.
Body Weight	Negative:	Overweight runs in the family. I can't buck heredity.
	Positive:	Small permanent changes in eating and exercise habits make a large difference in weight loss. I will be patient in waiting for the results.
Food Pattern	Negative:	I like junk food. The cholesterol theory is controversial; who knows what to believe these days.
	Positive:	Food preferences are acquired. I can lower my intake of saturated fat, cholesterol, sugar, and salt and still eat foods I enjoy.
Stress Management	Negative:	There's nothing I can do about the stresses I face every day. I am high-strung and can't change that.
	Positive:	I want to learn how to control my responses to stress; my life would be more pleasant and productive if I didn't lose so much energy responding ineffectively to stress.

Although all of us talk to ourselves, we do not habitually pay close attention to what we say. Monitoring your self-talk will reveal initial barriers to change that need to be overcome. Record examples of inner monologues during this period.

If you tell yourself you are going to, let us say, increase your level of physical activity, what thoughts come to mind? Do you automatically say to yourself things like "What a nuisance" or "I really don't have time for this"? If negative thoughts do spontaneously come to mind, work to overcome them by substituting positive responses in their place—for example, "I'll have more energy and will feel refreshed if I take a brisk walk before dinner."

Record these negative and positive inner monologues in a small notebook that you carry with you. Keep all your behavior change information in this notebook. Although record keeping may seem bothersome at first, it is an extremely important part of achieving long-term behavior changes. This preliminary self-observation phase will prepare you for the more elaborate and detailed self-observation that will be needed during your active change program.

In this initial phase, you are making a conscious decision to expend effort to achieve long-term goals; you should expect some short-term discomforts and annoyances. Many habits are deep-rooted and they can't be altered overnight. The methods set forth in this book equip you with techniques that will bring about behavior change and make "relapse" less likely. But your own sustained effort is required, especially during these early stages.

TWO: BUILDING CONFIDENCE AND COMMITMENT TO CHANGE

Once you are armed with the first level of data and awareness of the problem, build your commitment and confidence for your forth-

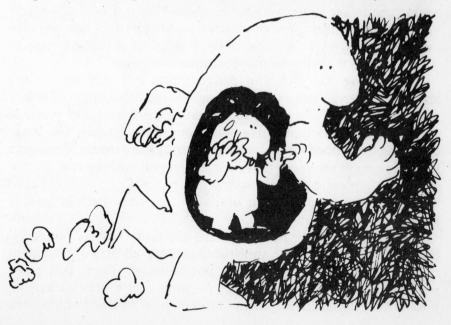

coming efforts. The neophyte exerciser, for instance, finds that parking the car a bit farther from the office provides exercise without much effort; the person who is cutting down on foods high in fat and sugar finds that two slices of bacon readily supplant the usual three; and the individual embarking on a stress management program discovers that a short walk calms his nerves as effectively as a drink does. These experiences start to build confidence and initiate you to the one-step-at-a-time approach that underlies effective behavior change.

Continuing efforts to deal with negative self-monologues will also aid you in building commitment and confidence that change is possible and desirable. Therefore, it is useful to make a plan to substitute helpful or positive self-talk for your previously identified negative and self-defeating self-statements; record these positive self-statements at least twice daily for a week or two.

THREE: INCREASING AWARENESS OF BEHAVIOR PATTERNS

Planning your program for behavior change often requires more elaborate information than the examples mentioned thus far. You gain a further level of awareness of behavior patterns, for instance, when you gauge on a pedometer the amount you walk per day and divide that daily pedometer reading into miles walked in morning, afternoon, and evening, or on weekdays versus weekends. This will enable you to see when you are most inactive and how you might improve your routine. You can learn how to identify when negative self-statements, anger, tension, or depression act as cues that trigger such habits as smoking or inappropriate snacking.

In analyzing your behavior patterns, you not only learn more about the internal cues (thoughts or feelings) that may stimulate your behavior but also how to recognize the social and physical environmental cues that similarly influence your actions. The alarm clock rings, the horn honks, the light turns green—these are cues in the physical environment that elicit semiautomatic behavior. For the smoker, completing a meal, having a cup of coffee or a cocktail in hand, or chatting with a group of friends may be powerful cues that stimulate the urge to smoke.

The actions of other people (praise, criticism, advice, nonverbal behavior), as well as their anticipated actions, all play a prominent role in shaping and maintaining our behavior. There is a story, perhaps apocryphal, illustrating the immediate and surprising power of the social environment on someone who should have been

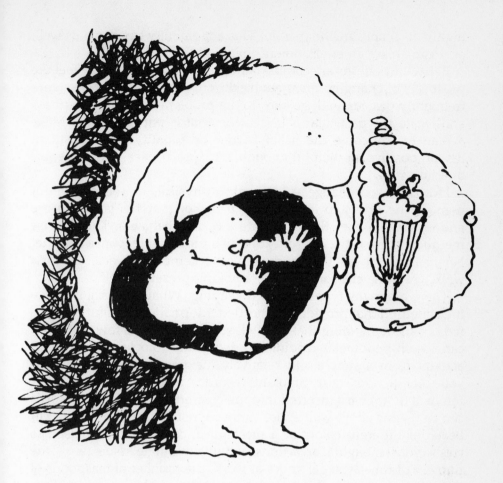

immune, if indeed anyone ever is. A university professor, a pioneer in behavioral psychology, was lecturing to his class about the influence of the actions of others on shaping one's own behavior. As he talked, he paced from one side of the lecture hall to the other. The students, having learned their lessons well, decided to use their own classroom behavior as a way to influence the professor's. Whenever he walked to the right of the podium, the students became fidgety and inattentive; when he went to the left of the podium, they sat on the edge of their chairs and nodded agreement with his point. By the end of the hour, they had him boxed in a corner of the room, oblivious to his predicament. Other versions of this story have the professor being induced to put his hand inside his coat in a Napoleonic stance, or describe how he, in turn, was shaping the student's behavior. Be that as it may, the point is the same: We are highly malleable and adaptable. This adaptability can serve us well, or it can create an environment that leads us to illness.

Behavior patterns are complex and, on occasion, you may feel the prospects of changing them are bleak. This is natural, but if you are frequently discouraged, go back to the problem-identification phase and locate the particular belief barrier that is impeding you. Make a plan to overcome the belief barrier by identifying a substitute list of positive or helpful thoughts to practice as a confidence-building step.

How can you change your mental, physical, or social environments? The first step in changing behavior patterns is to observe and record the cues that stimulate a certain behavior. Then devise methods to avoid the cue, or extinguish the usual response to a cue. For example, do not buy candy and other tempting sweets. Go for a walk when the cue for eating or smoking presents itself.

There are many types of record keeping. What is crucial is devising a method that provides the needed information without being so tedious or demanding that you will stop using it in a few days. You can obtain pedometer readings to determine your level of physical activity from a simple and relatively inexpensive instrument that you wear at your waist. Smoking records can be conveniently written on a 3″×5″ card inserted into the cigarette pack. Weight records can be posted above your scale. Various wrist-counters (with rows of beads of different colors or a mechanical counter) can be used to count your thoughts or actions about any single issue (e.g., the number of times you get angry at work, the number of teaspoons of sugar you use, etc.). Considerable ingenuity can be brought to bear on the topic. Come up with methods that *for you* are feasible. Moving pennies from one pocket to another as a way of counting a target behavior is a possibility.

Regardless of the methods of recording that you use, the important point is that you acquire the habit of self-observation and recording. Overcome any reluctance you may have to make this effort. Accurate self-observation is the foundation of your *entire* behavior-change program.

To make self-recording work for you, here are a few pointers. Your recording methods should be (1) portable and convenient (e.g., use a small spiral notebook), (2) available when the behavior occurs (e.g., if you want to count the number of times per day you become impatient or angry while driving, a wrist-counter allows you to do this without losing control of the car), (3) convertible into weekly graphs (if desired), and (4) reliable (but don't lose hope if you forget to record things occasionally).

FOUR: BUILDING AN ACTION PLAN

After further augmenting your commitment to change during a period of self-observation and recording, you are ready to develop and implement an action plan for specific change. The mini-change efforts described in previous sections have provided a warm-up for the sustained effort required to achieve major changes in one of your risk areas.

Your change program should be considered a means of problem solving in which you set a long-range goal (normally of six months' duration) and work to achieve it through a series of steps, each of which is preceded by a plan or self-contract of a few weeks' duration. The change is then attempted, the results evaluated, and a new plan is made for the next phase.

If at any time you reach a plateau and desire to coast for a few weeks without working on additional active changes, even that decision can profit from a self-contract to keep your change program alive. (If you fail to achieve a short-term goal, slip back a notch, or become generally discouraged, return to the earlier phases of problem identification and commitment building.)

Let me return to the example of a sedentary, overweight individual who has chosen increased physical activity as a goal. He has a pedometer, he has practiced his alternative list of positive self-statements, and he has identified sources of potential social support among his family and friends. His first action-plan contract could resemble the following:

TWO-WEEK SELF-CONTRACT: PLAN TO INCREASE AMOUNT OF WALKING

I will increase my average daily pedometer reading by an extra quarter mile per day, from my present two miles to an average of two and one-quarter miles per day during the two weeks of this self-contract. I will enlist the help of _____.

My responsibilities:

1. To focus on increasing my walking while at work, especially during my lunch hour.

2. To reward myself on each day that I reach two and one-quarter miles on my pedometer with 30 minutes (or more) of reading for my

own enjoyment. I will forego this reward if I don't reach my walking goal.

3. To record my data in my journal at 10:00 each night.

My helper's responsibilities:

1. To walk with me, when possible, during my lunch hour and to generally support my effort to exercise more.

2. To help me review the results of this action plan in two weeks.

Date: _____ Signed: _____

Review Date: _____ Helper: _____

This self-contract incorporates various principles of self-directed change, which I will now explain. You will likely wonder whether an elaborate plan is needed for a goal as minor as increasing the amount you walk by a quarter-mile a day. Although this first-step action plan may seem elaborate, it illustrates the important of *seeking small gains with good preparation*. Remember, too, that avoiding initial failure will facilitate further gains. The contract defines the action plan over a manageable short-term period.

Achieving Social Support

This plan engages the active support of a helper, because you are more likely to initiate and maintain a change if you have social support from friends and family members to augment your own efforts. Assume, for instance, that the helper in this action plan is a co-worker who usually takes some form of walk during the noon hour. This helper acts as a role model for the sedentary would-be exerciser. It is beneficial to choose an individual who can guide you in your practice of a new behavior. Both common sense and research experience tell us that helpers who have gone through a similar experience can be of special value. At times, however, you may need to create social support from fresh recruits to the desired change of habit. Risk-change programs can also be a family effort and involve several new "initiates." A word of warning: Not all helpers are helpful. Try to pick them carefully, and if you sense that their involvement is not working, then assert yourself and change to another helper or to your own unaided effort.

Self-Reward

The action plan includes self-reward, an important ingredient in self-directed change. The reward chosen by our sedentary friend (pleasure reading) is self-administered right after his nightly routine of checking his pedometer reading. Rewards work best when they are closely linked in time to the habit change in question. Thus, a daily reward for achieving a short-term goal is better than a delayed reward. However, adding a delayed reward to the program can provide an extra incentive (e.g., giving yourself weekly points toward a purchase that you are willing to delay until your point total has reached a certain level). The basic generalization is that the reward should be pleasurable, readily available, and (as in the case of the nightly reading) engaged in often.

The opposite side of this reward plan is, understandably, that you should be willing to do without the reward if you do not reach the goal. But your target goals should be ones that you *can* reach easily. Avoid heroic and excessive demands on yourself. Allow yourself to shape the new behavior gradually.

A self-administered reward can be either covert (a pleasant mental image or thought) or overt (going to a movie, etc.). Rewards may also be administered by others if agreed to through an informal or formal contract between you and a friend or family member. The earlier in the sequence of thought-to-action the reward occurs, the more likely it is that it will be helpful.

Generally speaking, self-punishment is less effective than self-reward. You can achieve results effectively without engaging in self-punishment. For some recalcitrant health habits such as smoking, however, the appropriate use of cigarette smoke itself as an aversive experience has proven helpful in quitting.

It is important to emphasize that self-reward methods, though they may seem to border on frivolous self-trickery, are surprisingly effective when combined with other methods of achieving behavior change. Many researchers, including members of the Stanford Center for Research in Disease Prevention, have found that self-reward is an extremely important factor in achieving permanent life-style changes.

FIVE: EVALUATION OF YOUR ACTION PLAN

Evaluate your progress daily during a risk-reduction program as well as at the end of each self-contracting period. Be flexible and willing to continue on the same path, to add a new goal, to change helpers if need be, and—this is of great importance—to return to the problem-identification and commitment- and awareness-building phases if you run into obstacles. Flexibility in cycling back and forth

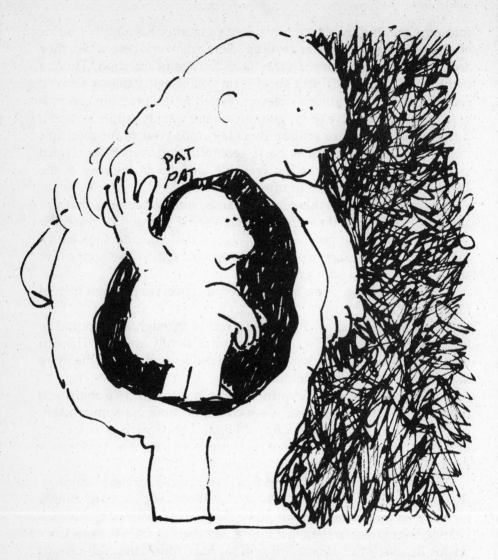

between the stages is crucial. You may have set unrealistically high standards. It is often useful to rebuild your commitment after a minor success by listing the unexpected dividends of your achievement. This is especially beneficial if you detect any faintness of heart as you devise the next stage of your action plan. Imagine, for example, that our would-be exerciser notices several benefits of his increased walking: (1) he discovers two new interesting restaurants on his walking route; (2) he is more refreshed and alert after breaking up his workday with exercise and finds that he has more energy, which enables him to accomplish his work more effectively; (3) he feels a sense of accomplishment from being able to begin to change his life-style by getting exercise at work (an activity for which he had previously maintained he had absolutely no free time available).

SIX: MAINTENANCE

As Mark Twain once remarked, "Quitting smoking is easy, I've done it hundreds of times." Dieters know well the frustrating cycle of losing and regaining weight that nutritionist Jean Mayer calls the "rhythm method of girth control." Successful maintenance of a change program is obviously of key importance. The daily effort needed for maintenance is less than that needed to bring about the original change. However, periodically returning to the methods used to achieve the change in the first place is helpful (e.g., the exerciser might wear a pedometer for a week every few months to refresh awareness of his activity level). Devise a monthly checklist to remind you to refuel your effort and commitment and to practice the skills that helped you make the desired changes in the first place.

You now have a good idea of your chronic disease risk status and know the basic steps and principles of achieving self-direct change. The chapters that follow will provide more specific ways to effectively lower your chronic disease risk factors. I recommend that you read these chapters in sequence. The stress management skills you will learn in the next chapter are necessary to carry out changes in all of the other risk areas.

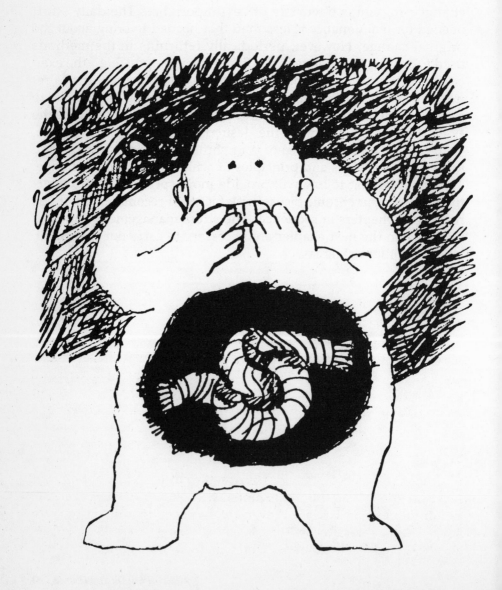

4

STRESS AND HOW TO COPE WITH IT

I f we were to judge by the number of television commercials about nervous tension, we would have to conclude that we live in a stressful world. The man with nervous indigestion, the frowning housewife with a tension headache, the harried businessman tossing about through a sleepless night, the apprehensive traveler reaching for a "calmative" are not characters in a play written especially for television; they are mirrors held up to a world in which stress is as sure as death and taxes. We daily confront ordinary situations that evoke stress responses, yet most of us simply do not know how to cope with stress. We have all had the experience of running behind schedule or feeling that we should have done better. Too often we overlook the ways in which we contribute to these common stresses by making unrealistic demands on ourselves and by responding ineffectively to everyday pressures.

Fortunately, we can do something about stress. And I don't mean taking a pill or an alcoholic beverage. Managing stress effectively is a *learned* skill—a skill that is of basic and vital importance to our general well-being and our ability to live fully and productively in a stress-filled world. With patience and practice, we can master stress management skills that will provide far greater control over how we react to the everyday pressures we experience.

Of all the risk factors in cardiovascular disease prevention, the most pervasive is stress. My experience in directing Stanford's Center for Research in Disease Prevention has been that if people learn stress management techniques, it becomes easier for them subsequently to make and maintain life-style changes in eating, smoking, and exercise habits. They find their lives more enjoyable. They feel better. The are able to accomplish more.

The mastery of stress management techniques is useful in helping not only to prevent heart attacks but also to achieve weight control and to stop smoking. Effective stress management can actually help to control blood pressure and may also help to lower levels of blood cholesterol (though diet, body weight, and heredity are more important controlling factors for blood cholesterol levels).

Although people vary in the ways in which they physically experience stress, most people feel muscle tightness, especially in the face or neck; a tight feeling or "knot" in the stomach or an upset stomach is also common. Much stress is experienced as a chronic, pervasive feeling of anxiety and inner tension. A less common set of symptoms—rapid pulse, dry mouth, and sweaty palms—is sometimes felt in response to specific, abrupt, and more startling stresses.

Despite the differences in cause, stress and anxiety responses do share a common underlying set of changes in body chemistry: increases in blood levels of lactate (a substance derived from muscle contraction) and of adrenalin and noradrenalin (hormones released during stress and activity that speed up the heart rate and constrict blood vessels). In fact, scientists have found that by injecting these substances into the bloodstream, they can simulate the physiological mechanisms triggered by chronic stress and tension and the resulting changes, both physical (increased blood pressure and pulse rate) and emotional (nervousness, irritability).

The most important effect stress has on the body is that it contributes to high blood pressure. This is significant to general health and well-being because high blood pressure is one of the three major causes of atherosclerosis. Learning to manage stress more effectively and thereby lower stress and tension levels thus serves a threefold purpose: It directly decreases some of the risk of having a heart attack or stroke; it indirectly assists you in lowering cardiovascular risk by helping you alter eating, drinking, smoking, and exercise habits that lead to atherosclerosis; and it provides you with greater personal control over your emotional and physical well-being.

An effective stress management program has six basic stages: (1) identifying the problem; (2) building confidence and commitment to change; (3) developing an awareness of stress sources and responses; (4) developing and implementing a stress management action plan; (5) evaluating the plan; and (6) maintaining the gains in effective stress management.

ONE: IDENTIFYING STRESS PROBLEMS

The first step in learning stress management techniques is to identify the kinds of stresses you experience in your everyday life, how these stresses affect you, how they depend on your physical and social environment, and how they relate to your own thinking. Once you identify the stresses that could benefit from better management, you are ready to make a realistic commitment to yourself (and to others) to change. Begin to identify your general stress level and your problem areas in stress management by taking the simple self-scoring test that follows:

SIMPLIFIED SELF-SCORING TEST
FOR GAUGING STRESS AND TENSION LEVELS

(Circle the appropriate number in each item)

Behavior	Often	A few times a week	Rarely
1. I feel tense, anxious, or have nervous indigestion.	2	1	0
2. People at work/home make me feel tense.	2	1	0
3. I eat/drink/smoke in response to tension.	2	1	0
4. I have tension or migraine headaches, or pain in the neck or shoulders, or insomnia.	2	1	0
5. I can't turn off my thoughts at night or on weekends long enough to feel relaxed and refreshed the next day.	2	1	0
6. I find it difficult to concentrate on what I'm doing because of worrying about other things.	2	1	0
7. I take tranquilizers (or other drugs) to relax.	2	1	0
8. I have difficulty finding enough time to relax.	2	1	0
9. Once I find the time, it is hard for me to relax.		Yes 1	No 0
10. My workday is made up of many deadlines.		Yes 1	No 0

Maximum total score = 18.   My total score _____.

Zone	Score	Tension Level
A	14-18	Considerably above average
B	9-13	Above average
C	5- 8	Average
D	3- 4	Below average
E	0- 2	Considerably below average

All individuals but those in Zone E have something to learn about stress management. Nevertheless, all individuals, including those in Zone E, should have another opinion. Ask a friend or relative who knows you well to rate your stress level from his or her observations. Have him or her take the test on page 59, adapted from one developed by Dr. Virginia Price and used in the Stanford Center for Research in Disease Prevention. This "observer rating" of how you handle stress may give you some surprising and useful insights.

If the score obtained by your observer is higher than the one you reached, assume that the observer rating is more accurate, because it is often more objective. Both the self-scoring test and the observer-rating test are useful tools in obtaining information because they do not test identical components of stress. The self-scoring test covers a broad range of physical and cognitive aspects of self-perceived stress or tension. By contrast, the observer-rating test measures only the habitual behavioral traits of anger, impatience, and a sense of time urgency. These are traits ascribed to the so-called Type A behavior that cardiologists Meyer Friedman and Ray Rosenman, authors of *Type A Behavior and Your Heart*, have found to be more common in coronary patients than in individuals of the same age who are free of coronary problems.

These tests should bring you closer to an understanding not only of the extent of stress in your life but also of the ways it is produced. After you are armed with this self-knowledge you will find it useful to discover whether you have important barriers to change. Many individuals find that obstacles exist in their attitudes and beliefs about the possibility or wisdom of changing deep-rooted habits. After identifying your belief barriers, you can then alter them by practicing a set of rational counterarguments that will make you more open to change (see the chart, Thoughts That Impede or Promote a Willingness to Begin Change, in Chapter 3).

A few common belief barriers are "I'm too busy to practice stress management" or "I am nervous and high-strung and I can't do any-

OBSERVER BEHAVIOR RATING INVENTORY

Circle the number in the box that most accurately describes how often _____ engages in these behaviors. Use scoring system on page 58.

Behavior	Never	Seldom (once or twice a week)	Often (practically every day)	Very frequently (at least once a day)
1. Hurriedness: Eats and/or moves fast.	0	1	2	3
2. Talking: Speaks fast, in an explosive manner, repeats self unnecessarily, and/or interrupts others.	0	1	2	3
3. Listening: Has to have things repeated, apparently because of inattentiveness.	0	1	2	3
4. Worries: Expresses worries about trivia and/or things he/she can do nothing about.	0	1	2	3
5. Anger/hostility: Gets mad at self and/or others.	0	1	2	3
6. Impatience: Tries to hurry others and/or becomes frustrated with own pace.	0	1	2	3
Maximum total score = 18.		Subject's total score _____.		

thing about it." Ask yourself whether you have these or similar beliefs that will impede your progress in managing stress more effectively. If you do have negative thoughts about your willingness or ability to change, substitute positive thoughts based on realistic expectations. (A busy, time-pressured Type A personality can replace the barrier belief, "I don't have time for this," with the realistic counterbelief, "I will be able to use my time more efficiently and effectively if I don't waste needless energy spinning my wheels because of poor stress management. By learning to cope with stress more effectively, my life will be more pleasant, I'll be healthier, and I'll be able to be more productive.")

TWO: BUILDING CONFIDENCE
AND COMMITMENT TO CHANGE

Ask yourself whether you have sufficient desire to commit yourself to the effort needed to make a change. A strong commitment is vital to successful use of stress management methods. Many people find that self-contracts are a useful adjunct—a physical act (writing) that expresses their commitment. Self-contracts also help people define their goals. A step-by-step approach in setting your goals is best. Start with small, manageable goals upon which you can build. You will gain skill as well as positive reinforcement from these initial successes. Involving a friend or relative is helpful in providing social support and encouragement for your effort. A self-contract to get you started might look something like this:

SELF-CONTRACT FOR THE PLANNING PHASE
OF STRESS MANAGEMENT

I am going to work on a program of stress management and I will enlist the aid of _____ to support and encourage my efforts.

I will set aside the following days and times for planning my program and practicing stress management techniques:

_____

Date: _____ Signed: _____
Review Date: _____ Helper: _____

THREE: INCREASING AWARENESS OF
STRESS SOURCES AND STRESS RESPONSES

Training yourself to become aware of your own sources of stress and the ways you respond can be aided by comparing a set of ineffective, stressful responses with a set of relaxed, effective responses in two fictitious individuals, Mr. A and Mr. B. In reading the instructional drill on pages 62 and 63, try to imagine mentally—and to experience physically—the set of emotional and physical actions and reactions first of Mr. A and then of Mr. B.

This drill demonstrates effective and ineffective coping methods: Mr. A's pattern of reinforcing his maladaptive physical and mental responses; Mr. B's pattern of reinforcing his effective physical and mental responses. Although these are learned behavioral patterns, it is unimportant, from the standpoint of being able to change unproductive behavior, to trace their original sources. What is important is to learn new patterns of stress identification, preparation for stress, and techniques to handle the actual stress situation and the post-stress period.

Careful record keeping is the next step in becoming aware of causes of stress in your life. In a small, convenient notebook record the frequency of, antecedent cues for, and reactions to external environmental stresses (people, places, events, and physical agents, such as noise) and internal environmental cues (thoughts stimulating feelings of anxiety, fear, etc.). Start a daily stress and tension log and record this information (in an abbreviated form that is comfortable for you) for a period of one or two weeks. A sample log, used in the Stanford Center for Research in Disease Prevention, follows:

DAILY STRESS AND TENSION LOG

Date _____

Stress or tensions felt	Time of day	Where? Doing what? With whom?	Thoughts or feelings	Response to stress
1. Tight stomach.	7:30 A.M.	Getting ready for work.	Worried about being late. Frustration	Hurried more.
2. Headache, tight neck muscles, fatigue.	2:30 P.M.	At work, trying to straighten out a serious foul-up.	Frustration	Got angry with associates.
3. Heart racing, tense muscles, and tight grip on steering wheel.	5:15 P.M.	In car on way home from work. In traffic jam.	Anger	Tried ineffectively to pass slow cars.

After identifying general stress patterns revealed in your daily stress and tension log, other forms of record keeping are helpful for

ONE DAY IN THE LIFE OF MR. A AND MR. B

Potential Stresses	Mr. A (Stressed, ineffective responses)	Mr. B (Relaxed, effective responses)
1. 7:00 A.M. Alarm clock did not go off. Overslept.	*Action* Rushed through shaving, dressing. Left without any breakfast.	*Action* Called colleague to say he would be 30 minutes late. Got ready for work and ate breakfast as usual.
	Thoughts I can't be late. This is going to foul up my whole day.	*Thoughts* This is not a big problem. I can manage to make up the 30 minutes later on.
	Results Left home in a hurried state.	*Results* Left home in a relaxed state.
2. 8:00 A.M. Traffic jam caused by slow driver in fast lane.	*Action* Honked horn, gripped steering wheel hard; tried to pass and later tried to speed.	*Action* Waited for traffic jam to end. Relaxed and listened to the radio while waiting; later drove at his normal rate.
	Thoughts Why can't that jerk move into the slow lane? This infuriates me.	*Thoughts* I'm not going to let this upset me since there is nothing I can do about it.
	Results Blood pressure and pulse rate rose. Arrived at work hurried and harried.	*Results* Remained calm and relaxed. Arrived at work fresh and alert.
3. 10:00 A.M. Angry associate blew up over a staffing problem.	*Action* Was officially polite but non-verbal behavior signaled impatience and anger.	*Action* Relaxed while listening attentively and mentally rehearsed how to handle this encounter. Remained calm in demeanor.
	Thoughts This guy is a prima donna. I can't tolerate outbursts like these; I'll never get my work done.	*Thoughts* Beneath all his anger he does have a point. I can take care of this problem now before it gets more serious.
	Results Associate stormed out unsatisfied. Mr. A was too aggravated to take care of important business on his agenda.	*Results* Associate's temper was calmed. He thanked Mr. B for hearing him out. Mr. B was glad that he was able to take care of the problem.

4. 12:00 NOON Behind schedule.	*Action* Ate lunch in office while working. Could not find needed materials in files. Made telephone calls but parties were out. *Thoughts* I'll never get out from under all this work. I'm going to plow through this if I have to work through dinner. *Results* Made mistakes in work because of exasperation.	*Action* Went for a 20-minute walk in the park. Ate lunch in park. *Thoughts* A break in routine refreshes me. I work better when I allow myself intervals to relax. *Results* Returned refreshed. Proceeded with work rapidly and with fresh insight.
5. 11:00 P.M. Bedtime.	*Action* Couldn't get to sleep. Had insomnia for two hours. *Thoughts* Why don't I accomplish more? I am a disappointment to myself and my family. *Results* Awoke exhausted and depressed.	*Action* Fell asleep rapidly. *Thoughts* This has been a good day. I'm glad I was able to head off several potential problems. *Results* Awoke refreshed and happy.

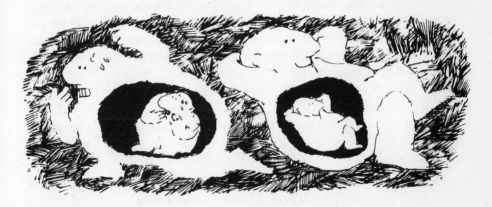

monitoring the frequency of particularly persistent stress problems. For those who are allergic to written record keeping, a variety of supplementary methods exist. You can use a wrist-counter when logging the frequency of a single type of stress stimulus or response. A wrist-counter can also be used to obtain an initial count of the daily frequency of a particular problem (e.g., feelings such as anger or frustration that act as stress inducers). After you embark on a stress management program, this initial information provides you with important before-and-after feedback on your progress.

FOUR: DEVELOPING A STRESS MANAGEMENT ACTION PLAN

The next phase in a stress management program is constructing an action plan for change. First, however, you will need to develop two basic skills, both of which are of central importance: deep muscle relaxation and mental relaxation. These skills are also important in helping you to bring about changes in your eating, exercise, and smoking habits.

Deep Muscle Relaxation

The technique that follows is one we of the Stanford Center for Research in Disease Prevention devised and have found most useful in our work. It is a simple relaxation method that incorporates elements of autogenic training, which originated with Drs. W. Luthe and V.H. Schultz in Germany and is used rather commonly in Europe. Though this is by no means the only effective relaxation method, it is easy to learn and practice. (Two points of caution are important: Under no circumstances should anyone taking blood-pressure-lowering drugs stop using these medications after starting relaxation training. You may find that your pill dosage can be reduced, but this should be done only in close cooperation with your physician. Furthermore, if you have a history of serious mental illness, do not begin a program of stress management without consulting your doctor.) Whatever time it takes you to learn these drills and make them work for you is time well spent. Do not skip them. With practice, the drills can enable you to reduce muscle tension; lower blood pressure; and decrease headaches, insomnia, and anxiety.

DEEP MUSCLE RELAXATION DRILL

1. Find as quiet an environment as possible. Lie on your back in a comfortable position or sit comfortably. Close your eyes.
2. For right-handed people, begin by physically tensing the right hand for an instant, then relaxing it and letting it go loose. Tell your hand to feel heavy and warm. Continue with the rest of the right side of the body, moving up to forearm, upper arm, shoulder, then down to the foot, lower leg, and upper leg. Next, follow the same

procedure on the left side of the body. (If you are left-handed, begin the procedure with the left hand and continue.) The hands, arms, and legs should feel relaxed, heavy, and warm. Wait for these feelings. After mastering the technique, you will not need to tense your muscles before relaxing them.

3. Next, relax the muscles of the hips and let a wave of relaxation pass up from the abdomen to the chest. Do not tense these muscles. Tell them to feel heavy and warm. Your breathing will come more from the diaphragm than from the chest and will be slower. Wait for this breathing change.

4. Now let the wave of relaxation continue into the shoulders, neck, jaw, and the muscles of the face. Pay special attention to the muscles controlling the eyes and forehead. Finish the drill by telling your forehead to feel cool.

Practice this drill twice daily; 15 to 20 minutes is ideal (but even three minutes is better than nothing when circumstances do not permit a longer session). Practice before meals or no sooner than one hour after meals. You can also practice before an anticipated stress experience but no more frequently than four times a day.

With practice you will learn to attain deep muscle relaxation—the feeling of heavy, warm, inert muscles and a cool forehead—in as short a time as two minutes. An Instant Relaxation Drill, which will be described later, is designed for use before and during stressful periods in the course of your normal activities when longer relaxation periods are clearly not practical.

If you are not sure whether or not you are relaxed during this drill, ask another person to raise your arm or leg about six inches and then let it go; if it drops as a dead weight, your muscles are relaxed. Jerky resistance indicates that muscle tension is still present. The benefits of deep muscle relaxation are many: lowered pulse rate and blood

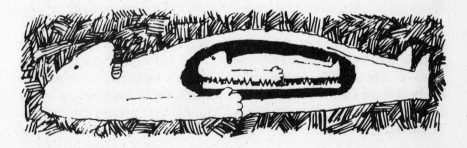

pressure, lowered breating rate, decreased oxygen consumption, and a general feeling of calmness and tranquility.

Mental Relaxation

When you have learned to achieve at least a partial state of deep muscle relaxation, you are ready for the next step in relaxation: clearing your mind of stressful thoughts and worries through mastery of the Mental Relaxation Drill that follows:

MENTAL RELAXATION DRILL

After entering a state of deep muscle relaxation, you are ready to begin the mental process that deepens the relaxation state. Your eyes are closed and your forehead is cool.

1. Enter a passive state; let thoughts flow through your head.
2. If thoughts recur, respond by saying "no" under your breath.
3. Imagine a calm blue sky or sea or any blue area or object without detail (with your eyes closed). Try to see the color blue (which has been found to be a particularly relaxing color).
4. Become aware of your slow, natural breathing. Follow each breath as you inhale and exhale.
5. If you still do not feel calm and rested, you may find it helpful to use a repeated, soothing word (such as "love" or "God") or a less symbolic word (such as "now" or "breath"). If you find that using a word distracts you, try a sound (such as "ah"). Think of the word or sound silently, preferably during exhalation. Always remind yourself to keep the muscles of the face, eyes, and forehead loose; and to keep your forehead cool.

The Deep Muscle Relaxation and Mental Relaxation Drills are interactive and should ordinarily be done together. Once you have learned both drills, simply combine them. Practice this combined Deep Muscle Relaxation/Mental Relaxation Drill twice daily.

In our stress management classes in the Stanford Center for Research in Disease Prevention, we have found that using the Deep Muscle Relaxation/Mental Relaxation Drill as few as three times per week, combined with occasional use of an instant relaxation method (to be described), is sufficient to produce a significant lowering of blood pressure in most patients. Among that group, those who practiced the relaxation techniques most regularly achieved the greatest benefits. Other research workers in this country and in England have also reported beneficial results in treating high blood pressure through the use of relaxation methods.

In the beginning, until these skills are mastered, frequent practice is the best plan. It may take you a few weeks to lower your blood pressure and achieve the general feeling of relaxation and control that you gain from better stress management.

Imagery Training. Imagery training is a useful method to assist you in the Deep Muscle Relaxation/Mental Relaxation Drill. Imagery training breaks down mental blocks to the use of your imagination. For people who are out of touch with their bodies, deep muscle relaxation is sometimes difficult to learn. Test yourself. Think of your left ear and make it feel warm; then imagine your right calf muscle as feeling warm and heavy. Next try two harder tests. Imagine that your left leg is heavier than the right leg; then reverse the feeling. If you can do these tests easily, you should find it relatively easy to achieve deep muscle relaxation. If you cannot, you will benefit from the following Muscle-Finding Drill:

DRILL FOR MUSCLE FINDING

1. Lie comfortably on your back in a quiet room. Become passive.
2. Tense all the muscles of your body for about five seconds; then let them go as limp as you can. Notice the difference in feeling.
3. Repeat Step 2, but now exhale your breath slowly during the total body relaxation. This will help create a limp, relaxed state.
4. Try tensing and "letting go" of individual sets of muscles: hand, foot, arm, lower leg, upper leg, buttocks, neck, jaws, mouth, face, and forehead.

After a few weeks' practice, almost everyone will be able to reduce muscle tension significantly. If you are still unable to reduce muscle tension (even after a hot bath), you might consider consulting a clinical psychologist trained in the use of deep muscle relaxation or equipped to use a muscle biofeedback apparatus as a training device. When used by qualified practitioners, biofeedback techniques can be effective. Nevertheless, it has been my experience that deep muscle relaxation can almost always be achieved without resorting to such expensive and time-consuming methods. Relaxation tapes for home playing may be helpful for those who have difficulty with unaided self-instruction; taping your own instructions for these drills may also be useful.

Even when you achieve deep muscle relaxation, intrusive, racing thoughts may prevent you from reaching a stage of complete muscle *and* mental relaxation. You may find this stage of partial deep muscle relaxation and free association of ideas rather pleasant; it can be a time for surprisingly effective problem solving. To achieve complete mental relaxation, it is helpful to incorporate imagery training into your combined relaxation drill by following these steps:

IMAGERY DRILL FOR MENTAL RELAXATION

1. Bring yourself as deeply into the deep muscle relaxation/mental relaxation state as possible. Assuming that intrusive or racing thoughts remain a problem, continue.

2. Use the following two methods of "thought stopping":

a. When a thought returns too frequently or persists, say "no" out loud. If it returns, say "no" again. Repeat this self-command over a five- to ten-minute period, while remaining in the deep muscle relaxation and mental relaxation states.

b. If the verbal commands to stop seem to decrease the frequency of the recurrent intrusions, then change to a silent "no" when an unwanted, recurrent, or persistent thought prevents your entry into complete mental relaxation. When a further reduction in active thinking occurs, you are ready to continue.

3. Imagine a pleasant scene, such as a mountain lake, a calm ocean, a blue sky with drifting white clouds. Focus on this scene to replace the previous intrusive, racing thoughts.

4. When this succeeds, let the pleasant scene fade and enter the final stages of the drill.

5. Let a gray or black "nothingness" be the image before your closed eyes. Ignore any visual detail.

6. Finally, let blue colors drift in, often as patches. When they come, hold on to the particular feeling that lets the blue colors in. When you are at this point, you have usually reached zero muscle tension and complete mental relaxation.

Instant Relaxation. After you have achieved a satisfactory degree of success in deep muscle relaxation and mental relaxation, you should be able to enter partially into deep muscle relaxation and mental relaxation states within 30 seconds to three minutes. You are now ready to practice instant relaxation.

INSTANT RELAXATION DRILL

1. Sit comfortably. (You can also learn to do this while standing, such as waiting in line, or just prior to an anticipated stressful event.)
2. Draw in a deep breath and hold it for five seconds (count to five slowly), exhale slowly, and tell all your muscles to relax. Repeat this two or three times to become more completely relaxed.
3. If circumstances permit, imagine a pleasant thought ("I am learning how to relax") or a pleasant scene (a calm lake, a mountain stream, etc.).

Develop cueing systems to remind yourself to use this drill (for example, whenever you become impatient over having to wait). The Instant Relaxation Drill takes from 30 to 60 seconds. In most stress circumstances, you can benefit from using either a Deep Muscle Relaxation/Mental Relaxation Drill or an Instant Relaxation Drill. Each can be used when you are consciously attacking a specific, recurrent stress that you have identified. Each can also be used effectively as a refresher interspersed in your daily routine.

The skills you have learned for more effective stress management—problem identification, commitment to change, stress awareness, self-observation, relaxation and imagery techniques—can equip you to construct a stress management program based on your own needs. Initial goals will vary widely, but it is important that you progress with small, incremental steps. Plan your program for a week or two at a time. Begin with the once-daily practice of the Deep Muscle Relaxation/Mental Relaxation Drill. This drill will act as a genuine antidote for unpleasant effects of chronic stress and will decrease the likelihood of your reacting to many of the usual external or internal stresses you encounter. However, many specific stress-related problems may require additional skills that I will now describe.

First, let me give you a few specific guidelines on launching your relaxation practice. Earlier I recommended that you try to obtain social support in the form of a helper to assist you in planning your stress management program or to encourage you to stay with it. In addition to the support of one or more of your friends or family members, it is even more useful if you can enlist their active participation. Secondly, I advised you to create a self-contract to help increase your initial commitment to change. Rebuilding this commitment at key intervals along the road to effective stress management is *critically important*. Therefore, use self-contracts at this stage and at following stages, not only for the commitment they imply, but also for the specificity they give to your action plan.

An example of a self-contract for use of various relaxation methods follows:

SELF-CONTRACT FOR THE USE OF RELAXATION METHODS

I have decided on the following schedule for practicing relaxation methods in the first stage of my stress management action plan. My helper will be _____.

1. A 15- to 20-minute Deep Muscle Relaxation/Mental Relaxation Drill at 5:30 P.M.

2. Instant Relaxation Drills five times daily, at least three to be done while at work.

My responsibilities are (1) to practice the above drills as designated, (2) to record the number of Instant Relaxation Drills I practice per day, and (3) to place a small circular piece of tape with "R" written on it on the center of my automobile steering wheel and on the dial of my telephone as a reminder to do my Instant Relaxation Drills.

My helper's responsibilities are (1) to judge the extent of my degree of relaxation during the Deep Muscle Relaxation/Mental Relaxation Drill and (2) to remind me to carry out my drills.

Our joint responsibility is to evaluate the results of the program in two weeks.

Date: _____ Signed: _____

Review Date: _____ Helper: _____

After you have developed a satisfactory degree of accomplishment in your daily practice of relaxation skills (and *partial* success is all you can reasonably expect during the first month), begin your plans for solving the specific stress-related problems that you have identified in your daily stress and tension log. The remainder of the chapter will deal with these methods: behavioral rehearsal, self-reward, and stress avoidance.

Behavioral Rehearsal

A cognitive type of behavioral rehearsal was pioneered by psychologist Dr. Donald Meichenbaum. It involves first mentally imagining and then physically practicing a series of thoughts and actions concerning stress in order to improve your ability to cope with it. Behavioral rehearsal not only sharpens your awareness of what precipitates stress but also trains you to plan and use the most effective thinking strategies, self-instructions, and actions for coping with stress. (The "One Day" diary of Mr. A and Mr. B presented earlier is an example of a Behavioral Rehearsal Drill.)

For those who prefer to or must do these drills alone, behavioral rehearsal is usually effective without assistance, but it is well-suited for the active participation of two or more individuals. The Behavioral Rehearsal Drill, on page 73, provides an example of how to devise such a drill of your own by selecting a single, common stress-provoking experience or situation taken from your own stress and tension log. After you devise such a drill, create a self-contract or agreement in which you specify the times and situations when you will use the drill, as well as the goals you are trying to achieve.

Behavioral Rehearsal Drills following this format allow you to rehearse mentally the behavior you plan to use in preventing or handling stress. This is an active process and we of the Stanford Center for Research in Disease Prevention, as well as numerous other researchers, have found it to be more useful than mere passive reading or listening to advice without actual practice.

At this stage, you are ready to create your own Behavioral Rehearsal Drill and your own self-contract for its use. The duration of the drill and the frequency with which you practice it will be highly variable, depending on your initial success and on the complexity of your original goals. After your mental rehearsal, put your drill into practice in the real circumstances of your life. Your overall plan should focus on one problem area at a time, for periods of one to two weeks. Following satisfactory progress in one problem area, move on to another.

Monitor your success in application and your results to guide you in devising the subsequent stages of your overall action plan. Apparent lack of success can usually be traced to inadequate preparation; hence, in all phases of your stress management program remember to (1) identify the problem, (2) build your commitment, (3) develop awareness of the nature of your stress problems, and then (4) devise an action plan. It is extremely important to avoid a sense of failure; a willing "back to the drawing board" spirit is necessary. Don't set unreachable, unrealistic goals. Devise a program that you can follow and set goals you can achieve. To give your progress in problem solving a spark, reward yourself when you manage stress effectively.

Self-Reward

Although the use of self-reward may seem a very simplistic device, research confirms that adding this simple measure to a mixture of self-control tactics is highly effective in changing stubborn behavior patterns that cause undue stress and lead to heart attacks. When applying self-reward in your stress management plan, the following two rules of thumb are helpful.

One: Be as considerate of yourself as you are of others. Avoid overcritical, over-perfectionist tendencies. In our culture, we are taught to be humble and self-effacing. Most people need guided practice in using the self-reward of positive self-statements as a substitute for the self-punishment of negative self-statements. (Your friends and/or family members can give you important assistance in this area.)

To train yourself in self-reward, try these simple steps: (1) From the "One Day" diary presented earlier, note or list all of Mr. A's self-punishing statements. (2) Note or list all of Mr. B's self-rewarding statements. (3) Note or list all of the self-rewarding statements you can find in your own Behavioral Rehearsal Drill. (4) Make a list of your habitual negative self-statements or negative self-thoughts about your worth or performance. (5) If you can't recall any, monitor the occurrence of negative self-thoughts for a week in your daily stress and tension log (most people will have a list of five or six such negative self-statements or thoughts at the end of a week). (6) Now make a list of as many positive statements surrounding the same issues and insert these substitutes into a new Behavioral Rehearsal Drill of your own design. The positive statements of self-praise should be accurate; you should objectively be able to give yourself at least some measure of credit for the attributes in question. Here you must differentiate these instructions from vague positive-thinking admonitions of many self-help books. Identify specific negative and specific positive statements from your daily stress and tension log. It then becomes possible for you to use self-reward in problem solving within the previously explained framework of the Behavioral Rehearsal Drill.

BEHAVIORAL REHEARSAL DRILL

Stress-inducing Experience

Example: I am preparing dinner. I worked all afternoon, arrived home late, and am now behind schedule.

Sequence of Thought or Action

1. Becoming aware of the stress producer—specific thoughts or actions:
   Q. What thoughts or feelings tell me that stress is near?
   A. *Example:* I feel nervous, hurried, and I have a headache.
   Q. What thoughts do I have that are making me more upset?
   A. *Example:* I can't possibly manage this and have dinner by six o'clock. I can't seem to handle stress. I need some help.

2. Preparing for the stress producer—specific thoughts or actions:
   Q. What can I do to change the situation?
   A. *Example:* I will practice an abbreviated Deep Muscle Relaxation/Mental Relaxation Drill before I start preparing dinner. I will turn on soothing music at 5:30 and will make some low-calorie snacks. I will assign tasks to helpers ahead of time. I will tell everyone dinner will be at 6:30.

3. Handling the stressful period—specific thoughts or actions:
   Q. What can I say to myself or do that will keep me relaxed?
   A. *Example:* I can anticipate, prepare for, and prevent some of my daily stress. I can get others to help. I can use Instant Relaxation Drills if stress creeps in. I can imagine relaxing things (e.g., a waterfall) while I am doing routine things.

4. Following through after the stressful period—specific thoughts or actions:
   Q. How can I learn from the experience and how can I maintain my progress?
   A. *Example:* I learned that I can prevent counterproductive stress reactions. I did a good job. I am going to ask my spouse to congratulate me when this happens. I will reward myself by setting aside time for pleasure reading later this evening.

Two: Build self-reward into your Behavioral Rehearsal Drill. The use of self-praise before, during, or after a stressful experience is a simple self-instruction to set in motion if practiced in the context of behavioral rehearsal. You will notice that the Behavioral Rehearsal Drill is composed of four stages: (1) becoming aware of the stress producer; (2) preparing for the stress producer; (3) handling the stressful period; (4) managing the post-stress period. Self-reward can be used in all but the first stage. Examples follows:

Preparing for the Stress Producer. The fictitious person in the example given in the Behavioral Rehearsal Drill employed a Deep Muscle Relaxation/Mental Relaxation Drill before entering the pre-dinner hour and followed this with a half-hour of soothing music that was concurrent with the anticipated stress. Because both of these actions were overt as well as pleasant, they properly belong in the category of overt self-rewards.

The conventional wisdom that "cooling down" before a stress situation helps avoid a stressful reaction is accurate. This is supported by research that shows that the body's production of adrenalin and noradrenalin falls after deep muscle relaxation and mental relaxation and that one's reaction to stress varies according to the amount of these hormones the body contains.

Handling the Stressful Period. Our fictitious person planned self-reward with an Instant Relaxation Drill and with imagined pleasant scenes. Another example of a self-reward would be the use of self-praise for handling stress effectively during the stressful period.

Managing the Post-stress Period. In the Behavioral Rehearsal Drill, the fictitious person used self-reward by making statements of self-praise, by planning to ask for praise from the spouse as a reward for a successful experience in coping with stress, and by setting aside time for pleasurable reading later in the evening.

Self-contracts that specify the conditions under which self-reward is to be received as well as the specific nature of the reward are very appropriate in changing recalcitrant behavior and can be used effectively in instances where the Behavioral Rehearsal Drill has shown that an overt external reward is necessary to help overcome the problem.

Training in Stress Avoidance Methods

Avoiding needless stress is a learnable skill—a skill that involves environmental planning. This simply refers to methods of rearranging your environment to decrease the frequency of exposure to particularly stress-provoking situations.

Stress avoidance training applies not only to our physical and social environments but also to our mental environments. Our own thinking processes can act as powerful stress-inducing agents. Stress avoidance, although simple in concept, requires considerable practice to master as a skill. Again, as with other stress management skills, you gain this practice first by identifying the stressful cues in your daily life (revealed in your daily stress and tension log), then by choosing and developing for yourself a Behavioral Rehearsal Drill that is devoted to working on a group of problems that lends itself to environmental planning.

Special Problems in Stress Management

Stress cannot always be readily avoided. Sources of stress particularly apt to require special attention are those that originate within our own thinking processes. For example, suppose that Mr. A in our one-day diary has begun a stress management program. Say he has chosen as a goal decreasing the frequency of biased, highly critical, hostile thoughts that he has about the performance of various people he encounters in his daily routine. The following account shows how Mr. A progressed in his handling of this problem. Use this as a prototype for your own efforts to avoid needless stress.

Mr. A proceeded beyond a one-day diary to recording a stress and tension log for a period of two weeks. Inspection of the log revealed that frequent feelings of anger and frustration and negative self-appraisals seemed to occur largely at work. These episodes most often followed extremely critical thoughts about others. He determined that such thoughts were often unwarranted overreactions. Furthermore, he identified these critical thoughts and ruminations as stress-producing agents that resulted in subsequent feelings of anger, frustration, and discouragement.

He formulated a plan which provides an example of how to solve special problems that arise in stress management. In Phase I of his plan he simply kept a log of the frequency, time of day, and circumstances that preceded his feelings of anger, frustration, and discouragement. The resulting log confirmed his impression that the distinct episodes often occurred after he had engaged in negative thinking about others. (Mr. A found that he also engaged in negative thinking about himself and determined that he placed unrealistic expectations on himself and was therefore frequently disappointed.) His log further showed that the episodes of anger, frustration, and discouragement occurred most often in the afternoons, during periods when he experienced many conflicting demands on his time. In

Phase II he developed this plan to alter his ineffective management of stress:

SELF-CONTRACT FOR SPECIAL PROBLEMS: PHASE II

I will attempt to reduce the frequency of counterproductive feelings, anger, frustration, and discouragement at work through the following methods:

1. I will engage in a 10-minute Deep Muscle Relaxation Drill in my office at noon, before lunch. I will put an "R" stamp on my "In" box and on the refrigerator at home as a reminder.

2. When I feel rushed, and just before any potentially stressful encounter, I will use an Instant Relaxation Drill.

3. I will record the frequency of my episodes of anger and frustration.

4. I will plot the frequency of my target behavior for two weeks before and after I begin this plan and will evaluate at the end of this period.

Date: _____ Signed: _____

Review Date: _____ Helper: _____

In Phase III of this plan, he added the following steps: (1) "I will make a brief list of 'substitute' positive thoughts, which I will review every noon after my relaxation drill"; (2) "I will use these positive thoughts in place of the critical thoughts I used previously." At the end of another two weeks, he again evaluated his progress and made plans to record and modify his frequent self-critical thoughts as his next project.

FIVE: EVALUATING THE STRESS MANAGEMENT PLAN

The review period at the end of each stage of your program (e.g., at the end of each self-contracting period) is an example of the evaluation step. Check your records to see how well you are achieving your goals. Be sure that you have not set unrealistically high standards or expectations. Unrealistic, overperfectionistic goal setting may discourage you and lead you to abandon your effort altogether. If you suspect that you are asking for too much, too fast, reformulate your goals. Accept the one-step-at-a-time principle of changing deep-rooted habits and devise goals that you can achieve. Your successes will reinforce your confidence and your effectiveness in bringing about more difficult changes later. Use your skills to devise programs that focus on special problems, and train yourself to bring your goals comfortably into your reach.

SIX: MAINTENANCE

You *can* be successful in effectively managing daily stresses by practicing the methods presented here. After you have learned these techniques and have made desired changes in gaining more control over the way you respond to stress, you will need to revitalize your program periodically in order to maintain your gains. The daily effort needed to maintain your progress will be less than that required to achieve the initial change. Your new habits should eventually become almost automatic. The continued use of many of them (such as the relaxation methods) is enhanced by the pleasures they bring. Nevertheless, especially under conditions of unexpected stress, it is important to return periodically to practice your most basic skills in stress management. You will still need to be willing to apply effort to solve new problems as they arise. It is helpful to create a maintenance checklist for your stress management plan. For example, you may plan to use the Deep Muscle Relaxation/Mental Relaxation Drill only once daily and the Instant Relaxation Drill from five to ten times daily. You may wish to continue on a particular stress avoidance, behavioral rehearsal, or self-reward plan. All of these can be specified on a checklist for ready reference.

Through regular practice of these stress management skills, you will be able to achieve a degree of relaxation and control over the daily stresses you experience that can never be found in that all-too-often-used panacea—a pill or a highball.

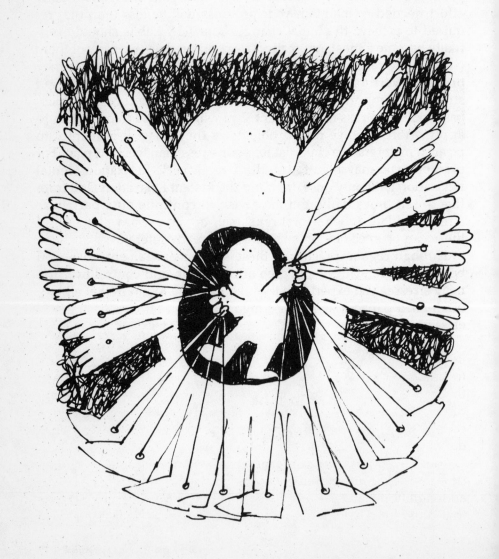

5

EXERCISE

For thousands of years man's everyday existence—even his survival—required physical exertion. The Industrial Revolution and ever-increasing automation has changed that. We have become sedentary to a degree that was never before possible. In the last 30 to 50 years, in highly industrialized countries physical inactivity among the bulk of the population has become the rule, not the exception. Today we must plan to achieve the exercise that once was an automatic part of daily living.

Think of children at play—running and jumping, climbing on jungle gyms, or playing ball. Children derive endless pleasure from their play; their enjoyment is instinctive and natural. Yet somewhere between childhood and adulthood, most Americans suppress their need for physical exercise and slip into relative inactivity, with occasional spurts of strenuous physical activity jammed into weekends or vacations.

Exercise is necessary for good health. We need to use our bodies in order to prevent physical atrophy. Whatever your present attitude toward exercise, I can assure you that your life will be enhanced through prudent, regular, and systematic use of your body. You will discover a greater sense of well-being, far greater energy, and a calmer, more relaxed attitude toward the pressures you experience daily.

Our need for exercise, unfortunately, contains a paradox. Once a person has become extremely sedentary over a long period of time and significant arterial narrowing has occurred, the very exercise that could have helped to prevent cardiovascular damage may present special dangers and must be engaged in with caution. Therefore, specific restrictions regarding exercise will appear later in this chapter. Do not disregard them.

Before discussing the types and schedules of exercise most appropriate for different age groups and, more importantly, how to use methods of self-directed change to achieve and maintain your new exercise habits, let us first examine some of the cultural roots that underlie sedentary living and the evidence that exercise is an important factor in preventing cardiovascular disease, diabetes, and osteoporosis.

Although some individuals truly overeat, *mass obesity* (that is, an extraordinarily high prevalence of obesity among a population) in the United States is due primarily to general physical inactivity. Americans eat less today than they did in 1900. Yet, despite this decrease in caloric consumption per capita, Americans weigh more now than they did then. Why? We use our bodies less. Hence it is only sensible that we attempt to increase our energy expenditure in order to get rid of excess pounds.

In an era when men and women engaged in arduous physical labor all day, inactivity during leisure hours was a reasonable cultural norm. Today, however, when daily work generally lacks strenuous physical labor, men and women need to devise ways to obtain regular exercise during their leisure hours. Yet generations of children have been brought up associating leisure with rest and inactivity. Consequently, we find people caught on both sides of the energy equation: We eat more than our sedentary bodies need and we are unduly inactive during nonworking hours.

THE EFFECTS OF EXERCISE ON HEALTH

Increased physical activity helps individuals control their weight through increased caloric expenditure, and vigorous exercise tends to suppress one's appetite, especially just after exercising. In addition, exercise helps to lower plasma cholesterol and blood pressure levels, producing further potential benefits in cardiovascular disease prevention. Two other major benefits of exercise are that it strengthens bones, thus aiding in osteoporosis prevention and in preventing or decreasing the severity of diabetes. Research studies indicate that people who increase their physical exercise are more likely to adopt other life-style habits that further lower both cancer and cardiovascular risks: They are likely to eat less, cope more effectively with stress, and even quit an established smoking habit.

Cardiovascular conditioning—which stems from an active schedule of regular, rhythmic duration (*aerobic*) exercise—results in many physiological changes that are likely to be beneficial in cardiovascular disease prevention. Aerobic exercise refers to sustained physical activity (at least 15-20 minutes) that increases the maximum amount of oxygen your body can process (i.e., deliver throughout your body) in a given time. Examples are brisk walking, jogging, running, swimming, cross-country skiing, and bicycling. Such exercise improves the health of your heart, lungs, and vascular system and results in a "conditioning" or "training" effect. Short bursts of activity do not produce this effect.

Aerobic conditioning brings about a number of beneficial cardiovascular changes. First, the heart's action becomes more mechanically efficient. The resting pulse rate becomes slower, and pulse rate increases after physical exercise or emotional stress are less than before physical conditioning. If physically conditioned, an individual whose arteries are already narrowed (an abnormality present to a moderate or even severe degree in many "apparently" healthy American adults) may be less likely to have dangerously rapid heart rates during sudden, unusual, or unexpected physical or emotional stress. (A heart attack is often precipitated by a rapid pulse rate.) Thus, physical conditioning, through its pulse-lowering effect, offers potential protection against heart attack.

The evidence in favor of this hypothesis is strong, though indirect. Two studies conducted by Dr. Ralph Paffenbarger of Stanford Medical School (one on San Francisco longshoremen and the other on male Harvard University alumni), for example, have indicated that vigorous exercise does provide cardiovascular protection. In these studies, Paffenbarger found that longshoremen engaged in heavy labor had fewer fatal heart attacks than did those who performed lighter work, and Harvard graduates who engaged in vigorous (aerobic) exercise had fewer heart attacks than their more sedentary colleagues. Differences between the physically active and nonactive groups were most marked with regard to the incidence of sudden death following heart attack. (About 40 percent of total heart attack deaths are sudden; the remaining 60 percent occur primarily within about 14 days after the attack.) Since most authorities ascribe sudden heart attack death to a rapid and ineffective heart action, the apparent protection experienced by the physically active individuals may have been partly linked to the lowered pulse rate resulting from physical conditioning.

There are other theories about direct benefits of exercise, but supporting evidence in humans is tentative. One longstanding hypothesis is that exercise increases the formation of new blood vessels leading to the heart, thus providing a natural counterpart of a coronary bypass operation. Another theory, based on observations of Dr. Paul Dudley White, suggests that regular, sustained aerobic exercise may increase the diameter of the large blood vessels. A third theory is that exercise increases the number of capillaries and hence the amount of oxygen that can reach the heart. These blood supply theories have received adequate experimental support in laboratory animals but not as yet in humans.

A fourth and more recent theory originated with a research team led by Drs. Peter Wood and William Haskell of the Stanford Center for Research in Disease Prevention. This theory suggests that some of the cardiovascular protection provided by exercise may be the result of beneficial changes that exercise apparently helps bring about in the distribution of blood cholesterol and blood triglyceride (the two main types of lipids or fatty substances present in the blood). Our group found that exercise sufficient to produce cardiovascular conditioning causes a slight decrease in *low-density* and *very-low-density lipoproteins*, which are the cholesterol fractions in the blood that have been shown to produce atherosclerosis in man and in experimental animals. This change was also associated with a large fall in plasma triglyceride levels since this blood lipid is carried in the very-low-density fraction. We had expected these decreases.

The surprising and more exciting finding was that exercise *increased* another cholesterol fraction—*the high-density lipoproteins.* (In the past, this high-density fraction was known to be, at the least, harmless in its effects on the arteries.) At the same time that our research group noticed this effect, other researchers discovered that this high-density fraction is associated with *lowered* cardiovascular death rates. Some researchers now call the increase in high-density lipoproteins in the blood an "anti-risk" factor.

Experimental work with animals suggests that high-density lipoproteins are responsible for scavenging deposits of cholesterol from various parts of the body, including arteries, and bringing them to the liver for breakdown and excretion into the bile. Therefore, the greater the proportion of high-density (versus low-density or very-low-density) lipoproteins in the blood, the greater protection one has against developing atherosclerosis. This seems to be an exciting new insight into the cause of atherosclerosis and may provide an important explanation for some of the cardiovascular benefits of exercise.

We have much to learn about the effects of exercise on human health. Still, the evidence strongly supports the thesis that exercise does provide a protective effect. We can also say, taking the lean and physically active Finns as an example, that the protective benefits conferred by vigorous exercise can be overwhelmed by having a high risk level in one or more of the "big three" cardiovascular risk areas (high blood cholesterol, smoking, or high blood pressure). The Finns' excessive butter, cheese, milk, and sausage intake raises their blood cholesterol concentrations, and their high salt intake raises their blood pressure to such an extent that the cardiovascular advantage provided by exercising and maintaining a lean body seems to be overridden. Thus, all cardiovascular risk factors are important; none can be ignored.

People can change sedentary habits—witness the vast increase in the number of devotees to jogging, running, bicycling, and tennis. If you already are a regular exerciser—a runner, a swimmer, a walker, a bicyclist, or a tennis player—then you know how exercise increases your energy levels. You know the satisfying feeling that follows exercise as well as the "below par" feeling when you miss your regular exercise. But if you are sedentary and are holding out with remarks like "I really should exercise more" or "I plan to start exercising when I am less busy," then you really do not fully accept or believe how much healthier you will be, how much better you will feel, and how much more energy and stamina you will have.

By leading a sedentary life-style, you are shortchanging yourself— allowing yourself to feel needlessly tired, overworked, and hassled by daily stresses and pressures. You are also adding to your (preventable) risk of having a heart attack or stroke. To change this situation, you can embark on an organized program to gradually increase your general level of physical exercise and your leisure-time pleasures involving exercise. This chapter will provide concrete ways for you to devise such a program, involving long-range goals achieved through small, incremental steps. *Gradualism* is critically important. Avoid the excessive zeal of overambitious efforts (too much, too soon) that are usually short-lived and are potentially hazardous. Do not try to remedy a lack of physical conditioning that has developed over a period of years with heroic attempts to whip yourself into shape overnight. Exercise should not be a physical punishment endured as a penalty for previous inactivity but a pleasurable, exhilarating activity.

Before discussing the methods that can help you bring about lasting changes in your exercise patterns, I will first describe the types of exercise recommended, who should use them, and for what purposes.

WHAT KINDS OF EXERCISE?

The two types of exercise I recommend are (1) general body movement for weight control and (2) aerobic exercise for cardiovascular conditioning as well as weight control. In the first category belong all low-intensity physical activities of daily living, especially those that involve walking. For many people, especially women who are overweight, general walking about that totals less than two miles per day is commonplace. This represents an *extraordinary* degree of inactivity. (Active working women and housewives often walk over five miles in the course of their regular daily activities.) Inactive people need to set a long-range goal (e.g., walking four to six miles per day) and work to achieve it over, say, a period of six months to one year. Gradual progress allows people to increase body awareness and fitness at a healthy, comfortable pace. Walking an extra four miles daily burns about 200 calories which, assuming there is no accompanying change in food intake, would result in a weight loss of about 20 pounds in one year. (This calculation assumes the extra walking is at the relatively slow pace of two miles per hour and that it replaces inactivity.)

Limbering-up exercises or calisthenics are also useful additions to a general exercise program. Neither calisthenics nor slow walking, however, has any appreciable impact on cardiovascular conditioning. To attain either the anti-diabetes effect or the cardiovascular protection cited earlier, you will need to engage in the second type of physical conditioning—aerobic (rhythmic duration) exercise of large muscle groups (particularly the legs)—to the degree that raises pulse rates to the levels stated below for various age groups (these are the pulse rates associated with achieving approximately 70 percent of maximum aerobic capacity). (See Table 5-1.)

Activities such as brisk walking, swimming, bicycling, tennis, rhythmic dancing, jogging, and running can all achieve this conditioning effect if carried out three or four times a week (on different days) for at least 15-20 minutes each time. Activities such as golf and bowling are not in the aerobic category. Your activity level should be

Table 5-1: Pulse Rate Goals for Aerobic Exercise

AGE GROUP	PULSE RATE	AGE GROUP	PULSE RATE
15-19	146	45-49	122
20-24	142	50-54	117
25-29	138	55-59	113
30-34	134	60-64	109
35-39	130	65-69	105
40-44	126		

sufficient to make you feel "almost tired" while exercising. To judge whether you are being sufficiently vigorous, after about five minutes of exercising stop momentarily and take your pulse rate at the wrist or the neck. Count for ten seconds and multiply by six. If your rate approximates that given in the table above then you are probably exercising at an appropriate level. As a further guide, you should be breathing heavily but still able to talk while exercising. Since pulse rates may vary ± 15 percent from the average levels given in Table 5-1, when in doubt rely on the "talking test" and the "almost tired" feeling to determine whether you have reached the appropriate level of exercise. (Alternatively, you may wish to have an exercise electrocardiogram taken while you walk or jog on a treadmill or while you ride a stationary bicycle; this will tell you more precisely what your target pulse rate should be.) Aerobic exercise should continue for at least 15 to 20 consecutive minutes at the 70 percent maximum level. Somewhat longer—about 30 minutes—is needed for brisk walking at a rate of three and one-half to four miles per hour. (The usual walking rate is about two miles per hour.)

A third type of exercise, generally called *resistive isotonic exercise*, is exemplified by weight lifting or pushups. Such exercise is generally useless for cardiovascular conditioning and is in fact associated with potentially dangerous increases in blood pressure. *Isotonic exercise*, in which one muscle group is forced against a resistance, is equally useless for conditioning but is not associated with as much change in blood pressure. My advice is to engage only minimally in these types of exercise and even that at a fairly low level (that sufficient to increase muscle strength to a slight extent). The lean, fit person who engages in a program of regular aerobic exercise is far safer in cardiovascular terms than the person working for muscles alone.

WHO SHOULD EXERCISE?

Almost everyone should be able to gradually achieve an average of four miles of walking a day while engaging in general activities. There are virtually no restrictions on general walking-about exercise save for those persons sufficiently disabled (for example, with arthritis) to make ordinary walking difficult or impossible. For these individuals, special rehabilitation efforts are in order and medical advice is clearly needed if it has not already been obtained. Swimming is sometimes possible even when the usual movements of walking are difficult. A stationary bicycle is often easier on the knees and ankles than is ordinary walking and may therefore be useful.

Before recommending a specific program involving aerobic exercise, let me spell out some special qualifications as to who is ready to engage in this activity. Many individuals have become so sedentary or have achieved such a degree of arterial narrowing, or both, that vigorous exercise may be hazardous. Such people should not abruptly embark on a program of strenuous exercise. Refer to the following "Readiness Gauge" to see whether or not you are ready to begin an aerobic exercise program. You may need to consult your doctor first and/or reduce other cardiovascular risks.

READINESS GAUGE FOR EMBARKING ON AN EXERCISE PROGRAM

1. Refer to the Simplified Self-Scoring Test of Chronic Disease Risk (Chapter 3, pages 38-39). If your risk score is above 13, you will need to have a comprehensive physical examination before embarking on an exercise program. Have your doctor confirm your self-rating of risk factors associated with salt intake (i.e., your blood pressure rating) and saturated fat and cholesterol intake (i.e., your blood cholesterol level). You may have scored up to eight points in these two categories. If your risk score in either the blood pressure or the blood cholesterol category (obtained as the average of *at least* two separate readings) is three points or more, then work to lower your cardiovascular risk below the three-point level before embarking on aerobic activity. If you are already engaging in aerobic exercise and have done so for some time, your physician may encourage you to continue.

2. If you are over 40 years of age, you should have a routine physical examination *and* an exercise electrocardiogram before beginning an aerobic exercise program or increasing your current level

of such activity. This is especially important if you have not had a physical examination within three years, if you have a family history of coronary disease, if you have ever experienced chest pain on exertion, if you have ever had elevated blood pressure, or if you currently walk less than two and one-half miles per day.

After gauging your readiness, you can now begin to devise your exercise plan. The six steps you will use are now familiar to you from earlier chapters: (1) identifying the problem, (2) building commitment, (3) increasing awareness of your patterns of exercise, (4) developing and implementing an action plan, (5) evaluating your plan, and (6) maintaining your progress.

ONE: IDENTIFYING THE PROBLEM

The first step in a program to increase your physical fitness is to assess your current level of physical activity. Use the Simplified Self-Scoring Test of Chronic Disease Risk to determine your risk score for physical activity as well as your total risk score. You can calculate your exercise-related cardiovascular risk from either a pedometer reading or a self-assessment of your physical activity based on the amount of aerobic exercise that you engage in regularly. You will need a period of at least two weeks of daily pedometer readings or monitoring of your aerobic exercise activity to insure that your rating is representative.

Most people will fall somewhere between the range of individuals who engage in virtually no aerobic exercise and whose pedometer readings are less than two and one-half miles per day (placing them in the highest risk category with regard to physical activity) and individuals with adequate pedometer readings (at least four and one-half to six miles per day) but with an inadequate amount of regular aerobic exercise.

If you find yourself within this majority group, improvement is needed. Take this opportunity to make a formal, conscious decision to increase your level of physical activity. A formal measure, such as writing a self-contract, can be important in getting you moving and keeping you going. (See Chapter 3, pages 49–50, for a sample self-contract on beginning an exercise program.) Reinforce your decision by announcing your intentions to friends or family and, if possible, enlist someone to help you in your efforts.

After you have made your commitment to change, you are ready to identify potential barriers you may encounter. Begin to locate such obstacles by keeping a diary in which you briefly record your daily activities and your attitudes about exercising more. Do this for a week or two. A sample daily activity diary might look like the Daily Activity Diary shown below.

This sample diary clearly indicates deficient physical activity. It also reveals the undesirable tendency to break out of sedentary habits with overzealous weekend activities for which one is not conditioned. This is often called the weekend-warrior complex. Keeping an activity diary allows you to focus on your thoughts about exercise and discover some of the clues to your inactivity; you will become more aware of excuses you make to yourself as well as of opportunities for regular exercise that do exist in your daily routine.

Some people simply settle into passive acceptance of a sedentary life-style, unaware of the hazards and lowered zest for living connected with physical inactivity. For such people, merely becoming more aware may be enough to get them started on organizing new activities and living more actively. Other people encounter distinct barriers in firmly imbedded self-concepts that exclude the thought of exercising more. Such people may see themselves as mature, dig-

DAILY ACTIVITY DIARY

Date: _____ Name: _____

Time	Activity	Thoughts About Exercise
8:00 A.M.	Leaving for work in car.	Could ride my bike or walk—don't have time.
10:45 A.M.	Leaving for a meeting a few blocks from the office—take car.	Everyone else is driving. I don't want to be the only one to walk.
12:00 NOON– 1:00 P.M.	Going to lunch and returning to office—in car.	Could walk but it's hot out. I'll drive and save time.
3:00 P.M.	Another meeting a few blocks away—go in car.	Feel too rushed to walk—will save a few minutes by driving.
6:00 P.M.	Going home—take car.	Maybe I'll take a walk this evening if I feel like it.
8:30 P.M.	After dinner, finishing some uncompleted work.	My neck is sore again and my back is aching. I'm too worn out to exercise now.
10:30 P.M.	Take pedometer reading before going to bed—walked one mile total today.	I just don't have many opportunities to exercise during the week because of my schedule. I'll play tennis for two hours this weekend to make up for this.

nified adults settled in a comfortable, sedentary groove and may feel that exercise is childish or for people more athletic than themselves. Let's look further into a few other rationalizations used to defend inactivity.

Too Busy. People who say they do not have time to exercise are generally making an excuse for the fact that they do not *want* to exercise. Exercise does not come high on their list of priorities. These may be highly time-pressured individuals who do not allow sufficient outlets for needed physical activity. As a result, such individuals can become needlessly tense as they internalize the daily pressures they face. They get out of shape and lack the physical energy that comes from regular exercise. Such people may become more interested in exercising after they embark on a stress management plan and discover how effective exercise is in enabling them to manage stress better. Since the "too busy" person is often a "Type A" personality, after losing some of his or her continual internal struggle with time pressures, such a person is often more willing and able to carry out an exercise plan.

Unaware. People who think there are few outlets for exercise in their daily routine may be overlooking obvious opportunities that do exist. Keeping a diary of physical activity can help people recognize and take advantage of possibilities for exercise.

Trapped. Some people who feel trapped by their environment have legitimate concerns about the safety of walking in certain neighborhoods. Solutions for this problem include daytime walking, the use of a buddy system when exercising outdoors, and engaging in indoor exercise (e.g., stationary bicycling or running, joining a gym or health club, etc.). Other people, including commuters, moonlighters, and parents of infants or young, active children, can feel trapped by having so little leisure time and so many restrictions on their freedom to use their bodies (modern American department stores, office buildings, apartments, and hotels often declare stairways off-limits to shoppers, workers, or residents, who must then use elevators or escalators for their vertical excursions). Another group of individuals in this general category are people who face significant social disruptions in their lives. Marital or financial problems, work-related anxieties, illness in the family, or difficulties with one's children or relatives often result in one's personal health being allotted a very low priority. With ingenuity, people in these situations can still discover outlets for exercise in their daily routines. It is critical that such individuals give their own personal health and

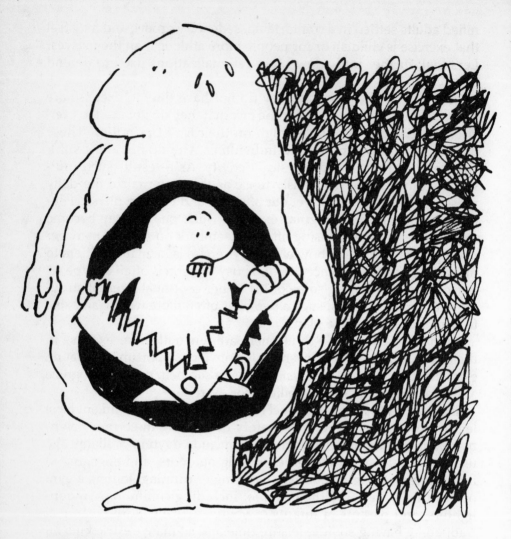

well-being the high priority it deserves. Some of the anxiety experienced by the "trapped" is often relieved by regular physical exercise.

Fearful. People who are fearful that they are currently not "fit" enough to begin an exercise program may have sound instincts. When unconditioned sedentary people overzealously launch new exercise plans, they expose themselves to the risk of potential bodily harm. Such people should consult a doctor before embarking on an exercise program and should achieve progress *gradually.* A small minority of people find aerobic exercise almost impossible and cannot attain a full six miles of walking. Such people can discuss with their physican what level of physical activity *is* safe.

Don't know how. Many sedentary people don't know how to begin. (What shoes should I buy? I have lost my confidence in my bike-riding skill. What do I do when it rains?) The remedy for this comes from the twin solutions of gradualism in your own attempts (for the sake of building confidence and for safety) and in learning from others. A visit to a sporting goods store and talking or practicing with sympathetic friends who exercise will be helpful. Comfortable running shoes or walking shoes are readily available (the best running shoes have an elevated heel built into them to decrease the likelihood of harm to the Achilles tendon). You can contact hiking or walking groups through organizations such as the Sierra Club. Your local YMCA and community college are excellent sources of information on classes in which to learn and practice new exercise plans, including weekend "Fun Runs" (a group activity in many parts of the country that has succeeded in getting the competitive aura out of running). The Age-Grouped Running Program and the Swim Masters Program for swimmers, sponsored by the Amateur Athletic Union, offer opportunities for people to join with others of their age in these activities. Your local high school athletic department or YMCA should be able to help you find out more about such programs.

Walking My Way by John Merrill is an excellent handbook for walkers of all kinds. For people interested in more strenuous mountain hiking, a definitive guide is *The Complete Walker* by Colin Fletcher. Both books give advice and inspiration that make walking a joyful pursuit.

Having explored some common belief barriers about exercise, you are ready to locate your own obstacles. From your diary, compile a list of your attitudes about exercise. After you locate your resistances, make a list of realistic, rational counterbeliefs. When you find yourself having negative attitudes about exercising, practice challenging these beliefs and substituting positive counterbeliefs. For example, when you say to yourself, "I'm too tired to exercise," tell yourself that a ten-minute walk would be refreshing. You may find it helpful to write a self-contract in which you agree to practice substituting positive statements to counter your negative thoughts about exercise at least twice a day. Soon you should begin to challenge the validity of your former negative thought *automatically* and become increasingly comfortable with positive attitudes about exercising more.

TWO: BUILDING YOUR COMMITMENT TO
AN EXERCISE PROGRAM

Once you have overcome some of your resistance to change, further build your commitment through a self-contract that states your intentions to proceed and to seek help from others. Talk with friends or acquaintances who are exercisers and ask for advice and encouragement. Such people can be very valuable in augmenting your desire to be more active and suggesting opportunities for exercise.

THREE: INCREASING AWARENESS OF YOUR
PATTERNS OF EXERCISE

Increase your awareness of your current patterns of exercise and of possibilities for incorporating exercise into your daily routine through careful record keeping that tells you more about the kinds of exercise patterns you have (or do not have). For example, if you are almost completely sedentary on weekends and are reasonably active during the work week (or vice versa), then you can identify the specific factors in your environment that need attention.

The following exercise diary provides an example of how a weekly summary of physical activity may be recorded:

WEEKLY EXERCISE DIARY

	Mon.	Tues.	Wed.	Thur.	Fri.	Sat.	Sun.	Total for Week	Average per Day
Miles of Walking About	2.6	3.4	5.2	3.2	2.4	1.4	1.6	19.8	2.8
Aerobic Exercise Minutes	0	0	0	0	0	15	15	30	

An analysis of such a diary can be the starting point for developing an exercise plan.

FOUR: BUILDING AND IMPLEMENTING
AN EXERCISE ACTION PLAN

Identifying exercise problems, building your commitment, and increasing your awareness lead naturally to developing a plan. Again, it is particularly important that you build new routines into your life in a comfortable manner. Such an approach will allow you to avoid physical harm and discouragement.

Your goals will depend on your initial self-scoring of physical activity. Readers who already are at a relatively high level (e.g., aerobic exercise two times per week) can readily set a long-term goal of achieving a full aerobic exercise pattern during a six-month period. (Readers will find Dr. Kenneth Cooper's *The New Aerobics, The Aerobics Way,* and *The Complete Aerobics Program* particularly useful guides that provide a scoring system—aerobic points—for various types of exercise such as swimming, jogging, tennis, bicycling, and brisk walking.) For readers at the lowest level of current exercise (two and one-half miles per day or less on your pedometer readings and no aerobic exercise) a reasonable goal would be to go from two miles of walking per day to four or five miles per day within three to six months of general walking-about exercise. Though this may seem to be a snail's pace, a rather major reordering of one's life is often needed to more than double daily walking from such a low starting point. Introduction of aerobic exercise can usually begin during the first six months of an exercise program, or if desired or necessary, can be deferred until the second six months. You can be guided both by personal preference and by your total risk score in deciding whether or when to embark on a program of aerobic exercise.

Let us now proceed by studying a sample exercise plan. Say that you have noticed that you walk very little during the weekend and engage in little aerobic exercise during the work week. You can set a long-term goal to increase your general body movement exercise (walking about) and plan to focus especially on weekend walking and exercising aerobically twice during the week. Your first short-term goal might be to increase your average daily walking by one-half mile per day. Be sure that the goals you set in your initial one- or two-week self-contract can be achieved comfortably and without inconvenience or difficulty. Build your program on small successes achieved gradually. A sample self-contract for the first phase of an action plan follows:

TWO-WEEK SELF-CONTRACT:
ACTION PLAN TO INCREASE WEEKEND WALKING

I will increase my weekend walking (as recorded on my pedometer) from an average of one and one-half miles a day to two miles a day. I will enlist the support of _____.

My responsibilities:

1. To look for opportunities for outdoor walking on the weekend (e.g., take a ten-minute walk before dinner on both days).

2. To look for opportunities for indoor walking during my weekends (e.g., help straighten up the house or do some household activity involving physical labor).

3. To place exercise cues in various places at home and at my office (on the telephone, refrigerator, TV, car steering wheel, etc.) to remind me to exercise and to practice positive imagery.

4. To practice a positive imagery drill (using images representing benefits of exercise) five times a day.

5. To record my pedometer reading in my diary each night at bedtime.

My helper's responsibilities:

1. To walk with me before dinner on Saturday and Sunday and to encourage me in my efforts.

2. To help me review the results of this plan in two weeks.

Date: _____ Signed: _____

Review Date: _____ Helper: _____

In devising an action plan, set long-range goals which you will achieve through small, incremental gains. For example, increasing your walking by no more than one-half mile every two weeks will allow you time to "digest" your gains and become comfortable with them. As you develop your plan, be sure to incorporate the following elements:

Overcome Pre-Aerobic Barriers. If your self-scoring test of cardiovascular risk and/or your subsequent medical checkup (including an exercise electrocardiogram) have indicated that you need to lower other risk factors before embarking on aerobic exercise, you will want to work on these other problem areas while you gradually increase your exercise at a pre-aerobic level. For instance, you may wish to work on gradually losing weight and decreasing your salt, saturated-fat, and cholesterol intakes. You may also wish to practice your stress management drills to lower your general level of stress and tension.

Use visual cues and imagery and keep records. Remind yourself to exercise by placing *exercise cues* in various places—on the refrigerator door, on the selector switch of the television set, on your car steering wheel, etc. An exercise cue might be a rough sketch of a person walking. Such cues remind you to avoid too much snacking or TV watching, overuse of the car, etc.

Imagery is another useful aid. Make a list of positive images that represent how exercise will benefit you (see below). For instance, an image of a healthier, trimmer you can serve as a reminder that each additional mile of walking per day over a period of a year can bring about a five-pound weight loss.

In the first phase of your exercise plan, practice these thoughts and images five times a day. Use small exercise cues as reminders. At the end of the second week, review your progress and make any needed alterations in your plan. In your phase-two action plan (the next one- or two-week period) you may decide to increase your weekend walking by one mile per day, which can be achieved by walking an extra 20 or 30 minutes. Again, use positive imagery as a stimulus to encourage you to exercise. Record the times that you exercise and your daily pedometer readings in your diary. It can be helpful to monitor your weekly walking, for example, and display your progress on a graph such as the one on page 97.

Consolidate your progress through self-reward. Build an ongoing system of self-reward into your exercise program. Use positive imagery, for example, after taking a walk or otherwise exercising. Further reward yourself by doing something you particularly want to do after you achieve a short-term goal. For a longer-term reward, you may wish to give yourself points for achieving your weekly exercise goals. After achieving your weekly goals for a certain designated period of time (e.g., four successive weeks), reward yourself by making a special purchase, going out to dinner at a favorite restaurant, or

---

POSITIVE IMAGERY: BENEFITS OF EXERCISE

1. You are looking at yourself in the mirror and see a vital, slim, healthy person.

2. Fatty deposits are melting away from your arteries.

3. Fat tissue is melting away from your now overweight abdomen.

4. You are walking up a hill with cool fresh air going in and out of your lungs; you feel fit and energetic.

5. Your body feels warm and relaxed—you are experiencing the pleasant afterglow of exercise.

---

the like. The important point is to reinforce your program by giving yourself both immediate and delayed rewards.

Use environmental planning. Exercise cues can make you more alert to your need for environmental planning. Arrange your activities in a manner that assures daily exercise (using your car less and your feet more). Think of various measures to make it easier and more convenient for you to exercise. You might need to get your bicycle fixed, for example. If you don't have walking or running shoes (and plan to start a jogging or walking program), buy a pair. If you plan to walk or jog during the noon hour, leave a pair of running shoes at your office or gym. Be inventive.

Integrate social support from friends and family. Encouragement from your friends and family can be an important boost for your efforts. If you enjoy company, recruit companions for your exercise activities. You may find colleagues at work who would enjoy walking or otherwise exercising at lunchtime. Working on your program in conjunction with your family or with friends or colleagues will reinforce your commitment to continue your program. Clearly, this can make exercising more pleasurable for you, and the sharing can lead to a valuable interchange of support and encouragement.

In sum, your success in improving your exercise habits and your general physical fitness will be dependent on your ability to devise methods for adapting the tools of behavior change you have acquired to solving the particular problems you encounter in your own life. It is up to you to make these tools work for you. They can.

FIVE: EVALUATING YOUR PROGRAM

At the end of each two-week self-contracting period, you will find a natural opportunity to evaluate your progress. At this time you should make a conscious decision whether to proceed to a more advanced stage or whether to return to earlier phases of problem identification, building commitment, and developing awareness. The decision is based on whether you have reached your current goals comfortably and/or whether you feel particular problems need special attention.

SIX: MAINTAINING YOUR PROGRESS

Improved exercise habits bring immediate intrinsic rewards. You feel better, you look better, you have more energy, and you are healthier. Thus, good exercise habits, once established, have a naturally reinforcing effect. Still, you will need to focus on maintaining

WEEKLY WALKING RECORD

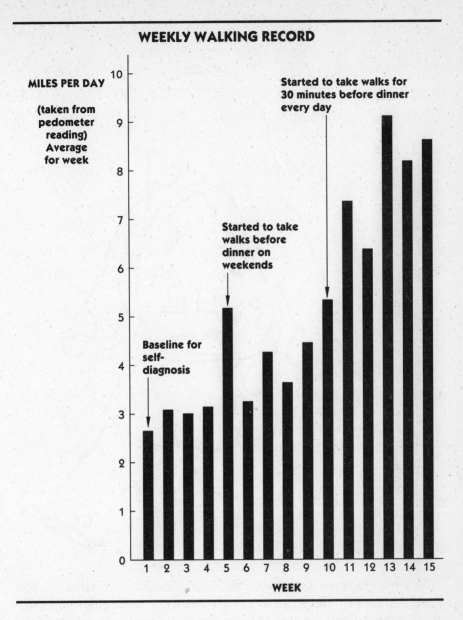

MILES PER DAY

(taken from pedometer reading) Average for week

Started to take walks for 30 minutes before dinner every day

Started to take walks before dinner on weekends

Baseline for self-diagnosis

WEEK

your new exercise habits. Periodically check your progress and work on special problems that you note. There are four general areas to review when working on maintaining your progress: (1) incorporating exercise into your daily life-style, (2) capturing the intrinsic rewards of exercise, (3) maintaining social support, and (4) monitoring your total cardiovascular risk level.

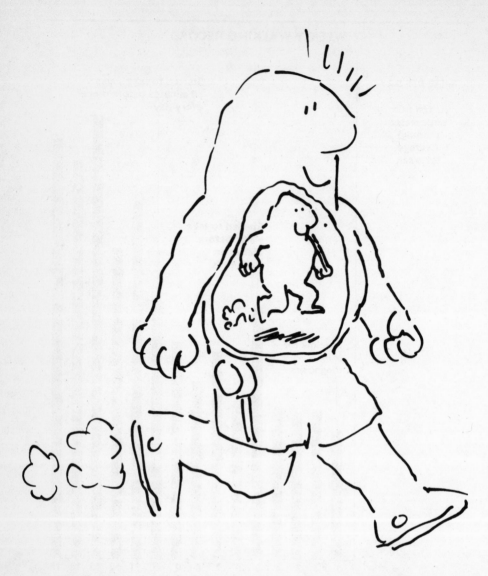

Incorporating exercise into your daily life. Check to see whether you have sufficiently developed ways to incorporate regular walking-about exercise and aerobic exercise into your everyday routine. You want your new exercise habits to become almost automatic. Seek ways to shop, visit, go to work, etc., by foot or bicycle. If you are a commuter, use stairs at work, walk to lunch, etc. At home, walking up and down stairs is valuable exercise. Periodically monitor how many miles you walk daily by wearing your pedometer for a week. Do not let your daily walking revert to previous levels.

Capturing the intrinsic rewards of exercise. Most people who have increased their exercise will experience a post-exercise period of exhilaration. For those who have not yet attained this feeling, I suggest that shortly after exercising you go to a quiet room where you have previously practiced your relaxation drills and attempt to tune in to your state of mind. Do you feel more content than usual? Become aware of sensations in your skin and muscles. Do they feel warm and tingling? Now practice calling up positive images that represent pleasant aspects of exercising. Think of feeling calm, relaxed, and exhilarated from exercising. Capture that feeling in your imagination and memory. Pleasant post-exercise drills can be used effectively as periodic rewards and as reminders of the benefits of exercise. If you feel sick, sore, or totally exhausted after exercising, you are being overzealous. Do not use exercise as punishment. Make exercise a positive experience.

Monitoring your chronic disease level. A periodic rescoring of your exercise-related chronic disease risk and your overall chronic disease level can give you important feedback on your progress and incentive to continue your program. A rescoring every six months is a sensible goal for a period of at least three years. Sound exercise habits will reward you in many ways and will automatically help you control stress and weight problems more effectively.

Exercise alone, however, is not enough to prevent cardiovascular and other health problems. The chapter that follows concerns food, a risk factor that critically influences your overall chronic disease risk. What you eat has a profound effect on three cardiovascular risks—high blood pressure, high blood cholesterol, and excess body weight. By changing and improving the kinds of foods you eat, you can do much to prevent not only needless cardiovascular disease and diet-related cancer, but you can also help prevent adult onset diabetes and osteoporosis.

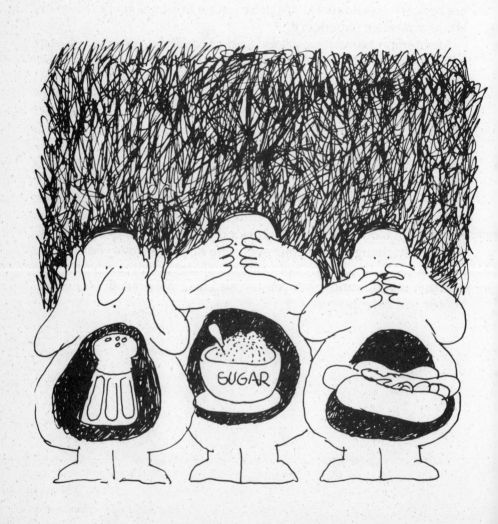

6

THE ALTERNATIVE FOOD PATTERN

Although you may automatically consider your diet to be a healthy one, your assumption deserves examination. The average American diet is, in fact, decidedly hazardous to your health. It increases the incidence of cardiovascular disease and all the diseases associated with obesity (including diabetes, gout, osteoarthritis, gallbladder disease, and high blood pressure), and recent evidence definitely relates diet to the incidence of certain types of cancer.

So much evidence for a direct effect of diet on the development of cancer appeared in scientific publications in the 1970s and early 1980s that in 1982 the National Research Council convened a committee of eminent scientists to review the evidence on the diet and cancer connection. The result of this meeting was the publication of a major document, "Diet, Nutrition and Cancer," and the conclusion was that dietary changes can indeed help prevent many forms of cancer.

Ever since the development of more efficient flour mills in the nineteenth century, bringing us white bread and with it widespread epidemics of vitamin B deficiency (because of the loss of vitamins and other nutrients during the milling process), we have experienced steady "progress" in food technology. This progress has now reached its apogee in a nation eating on the run, relying on the convenience of prepackaged, preseasoned foods, immersed in a sea of plastic containers and crinkly bags. The changes that have taken place are often too subtle to be apparent to most of us. For instance, white flour in the days of stone milling was not the present day ultra-white product devoid of vitamin E and fiber that we now get in our breads and cakes.

Pre-industrial man of course had his share of nutritional disasters. He suffered from periodic famine and a variety of deficiency disorders (goiter, for instance, afflicted thousands in iodine-poor regions of the world). Yet, on the whole, his sensing devices served him remarkably well. Food wisdom was passed from one generation to the next, and centuries of tribal learning resulted in a balanced, nutritionally healthy diet. Today we cannot return to the ecological simplicity of tribal man. If we are to cope with the challenges of the present and the future, if we are to feed a world population that will double in 30 years, we must in fact accelerate scientific and technological advance, particularly in such fields as animal husbandry, food storage, and plant genetics. Science and technology not only serve our pleasure and convenience, they also confer upon us vast opportunities—and with them a new set of responsibilities to determine what is a safe and healthy course to follow.

In the future we will need to increase greatly the amount and quality of health education in order to bring to everyone the nutritional knowledge that will enable us to reap the health benefits of science and technology and eat both healthily and economically. Fortunately, the prospects for an increase in this type of mass education are strong, owing to the widespread public interest in nutritional health. In this chapter, I will address methods for adopting a healthier pattern of eating. Because what I am speaking of goes beyond the usual concept of "diet," I call it an "alternative food pattern."

Before discussing this alternative food pattern, let me first examine some of the hazardous elements of the average American diet, specifically the problems caused by consuming too much salt, too much cholesterol and saturated fat, and too much sugar and high-calorie junk food. I will also describe the relationship of nutrition to cancer and will discuss common misconceptions about nutrition, such as the protein myth, as well as a cultural fetish—the rich-food fixation.

SALT INTAKE

The average American consumes 12 grams of salt a day, although many of us have recently shifted to lower salt foods. Medical studies indicate that this high salt intake contributes to elevated blood pressure. There are isolated pockets of people in the world, for

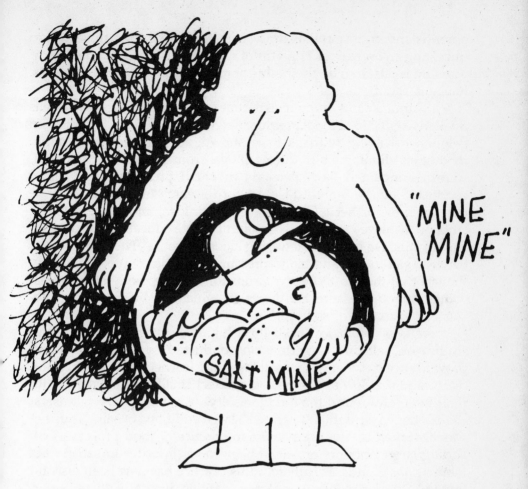

"MINE MINE"

SALT MINE

example, whose blood pressure levels not only are much below what we consider "normal" but also do not rise with age, as they do in the United States. Among these groups, very low salt intakes—one gram or less per day—are typical. Although other dietary or cultural factors may also play a contributing role, studies comparing ethnically similar people whose diets vary markedly with respect to salt intake provide further evidence that a high salt intake contributes significantly to high blood pressure. The people of northern and southern Japan, for instance, have a similar ethnic background and body weight. Both groups have salt intakes considerably higher than in most other parts of the world, but the average salt intake in northern Japan (about 40 grams a day) is double that in the south (about 18 grams a day). The average blood pressure levels of these two groups clearly reflect this difference. Similarly, studies of Solomon Islanders reveal that those who cook their food in seawater (ingesting an average of 11 grams of salt a day) have far higher blood pressure levels than do their ethnic brothers inland whose daily salt intake is about one gram.

Both animal and human experiments indicate that when salt intake is reduced, blood pressure levels tend to drop. Studies in Belgium involving humans have shown, for instance, that quite modest salt limitations (reducing intake from 11 to 5 grams a day) were accompanied by a decrease in blood pressure. In a study conducted by the Stanford Center for Research in Disease Prevention in two northern California communities, moderate salt restriction, achieved through a community-wide educational program, was an effective means of lowering blood pressure. The relationship between salt intake and blood pressure is further demonstrated by the fact that the most effective drugs for treating moderate degrees of high blood pressure are diuretics, which act by increasing the kidneys' excretion of sodium.

There is no biological need for a high salt intake. The excellent studies on salt and hypertension conducted by Dr. Lewis Dahl provide strong evidence that salt tastes are learned, not innate. Dahl discovered that low salt users could detect small additions of salt to their food (and found the food too salty), whereas heavy salt users did not detect (and thus "tolerated") large additions of salt. (Thus he was disturbed by the once-common practice of food processors of adding large amounts of salt to baby foods in order to satisfy the mothers' taste buds. Fortunately, this practice has now been discontinued.) Our desire for salt is highly adaptive. By gradually reducing our salt intake, we can increase our sensitivity to salt and wean our palates of the salt proclivity.

CHOLESTEROL AND SATURATED-FAT INTAKE

Cholesterol and saturated fat are somewhat more difficult to detect in the diet than is salt. The fats in beef, lamb, pork, and dairy products are highly saturated, as are those in coconut oil (used in ice cream substitutes) and palm oil (used in various processed foods).

Many fats are *hidden* in many fried foods served in fast-food outlets and in baked products such as croissants and various types of cookies and pastry. A visit to the kitchen of a fast-food restaurant would reveal large chunks being sliced off huge rectangular bricks of white lard or beef fat to be placed in the deep frying vessels. One picture is surely worth a thousand words after this experience.

Sauces used in restaurants are also another common source of hidden saturated fats. Except for palm and coconut oil, vegetable oils are predominately unsaturated. However, vegetable oils which have been "hardened" or "hydrogenated" by food processors also contain significant amounts of saturated fat. Animal fats in general are usually saturated, although fin fish contains highly unsaturated fat and the fat in shellfish, poultry, and wild game is considerably less saturated than that in red meats.

The unsaturated fats of fish have been the subject of many recent clinical studies. These "omega-3" fats seem to protect populations consuming high fish diets, such as the Eskimos, from some forms of heart disease. The result is that the Eskimos have a lower incidence of heart disease than populations consuming the same amount of fat from meat or dairy products.

Large amounts of cholesterol are found in egg yolks and organ meats, such as liver, which have far higher cholesterol levels than do other meats. Moderate but significant amounts of cholesterol are present in all meats, as well as in shellfish, fin fish, and poultry, and in dairy products (except for nonfat yogurts and nonfat milk). All foods of animal origin contain cholesterol as part of their cell structure. By contrast, cholesterol is absent from all foods of vegetable origin.

According to the American Heart Association, no more than 8 percent of total calories consumed should be derived from saturated fat (the current U.S. average is about 15 percent). High blood cholesterol levels are associated with increased heart attack rates, and numerous studies indicate that both cholesterol levels and heart attack rates increase proportionately as the percentage of calories in the diet from saturated fat increases.

In their outstanding "Seven Country Coronary Disease Study," Drs. Ancel Keys and Henry Blackburn found that high cholesterol levels corresponded closely with saturated-fat intake and, in turn, with the incidence of heart attacks and strokes in the countries studied. For example, the average blood cholesterol level of the Japanese, who had the lowest saturated-fat intake (about 3 percent of total calories consumed), was about one-half that of the Finns, who had the highest saturated-fat intake (20 percent of total calories) of the seven countries studied. The Japanese heart attack rate was the lowest, *one-tenth* that of the Finns, who had the highest heart attack rate.

Animal experiments demonstrate that by varying the proportion of high-saturated-fat and high-cholesterol foods in the diet, blood cholesterol levels can be raised or lowered. Furthermore, these studies show that not only can diets rich in cholesterol and saturated fats cause atherosclerosis (see Chapter 2), but also that a dramatic regression of atherosclerotic lesions can be brought about by placing the animals on a low-cholesterol, low-saturated-fat diet.

SUGAR INTAKE

Although humans have no innate salt craving or urge for fat, we do apparently have a strong natural desire for sugary foods. (Sugar, as used in this chapter, refers to *sucrose*, i.e., refined sugar.) Animals too, with the exception of cats, have a "sweet tooth," according to psychologist Dr. Carl Pfaffman of Rockefeller University. Technology, however, has allowed man's sweet tooth to be sated to unprecedented and distinctly unhealthy levels. Within 40 years after the first sugar beet factory was built in 1801, France was producing two pounds of sugar per person per year. Since that time, sugar consumption in developed countries has skyrocketed. In the United States today each individual consumes an average of 126 pounds of sugar per year.

Virtually everyone knows that sugar promotes tooth decay, but few people realize that a high refined sugar intake contributes to the development of heart disease. Refined sugar tends to increase triglyceride levels in the blood, whereas starch is less likely to do so. This may be because sucrose is more rapidly absorbed in the blood than is starch. When sugar reaches the bloodstream rapidly, it calls forth an increased amount of insulin from the pancreas, and the insulin in turn increases the liver's production of triglyceride-rich lipoproteins (very-low-density lipoproteins) which are associated with atherosclerosis. Individuals who are overweight, physically inactive, or who have a diabetic tendency are more sensitive than others to this sugar-insulin effect.

Sugar-rich foods are generally highly concentrated in calories and readily available in forms suitable for rapid consumption; both of these factors help promote obesity. When more than 10 or 15 percent of total calories consumed are derived from sugar (the U.S. national average is now 24 percent), nutritionally valuable foods are commonly displaced. Refined sugar has no nutritive value; it merely provides empty calories that appease hunger.

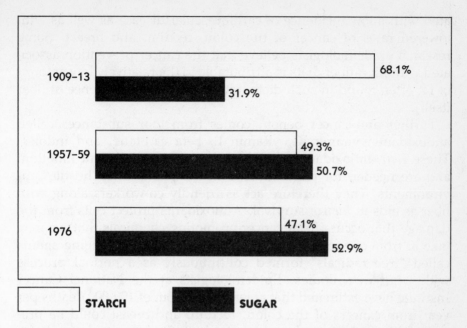

1909–13	68.1%
	31.9%
1957–59	49.3%
	50.7%
1976	47.1%
	52.9%

☐ STARCH   ■ SUGAR

Figure 6-1: Percentage of Carbohydrates in American Diet Derived from Starch and Sugar

Complex carbohydrates, found in grains and vegetables, are a common casualty of a sugar-rich diet. Complex carbohydrates once constituted a major and valuable part of the American diet, as seen in Figure 6-1. Unfortunately, starch and carbohydrates have fallen into disrepute in recent years because of popular fads, including "low-carbohydrate, high-protein" diets. In fact, complex carbohydrates are potentially the slimmer's greatest ally. Foods containing complex carbohydrates (common vegetables, rice, potatoes, legumes such as beans, unrefined cereal grains, etc.) as a group not only provide more complete nutrition (including balanced protein intake) than do refined carbohydrates, but also are lower in caloric density than are fatty or sugary foods; they tend to slow down the rapid intake of calories that often leads to weight gain.

NUTRITION AND CANCER

Another important dietary element often displaced by sugar is fiber—a varied group of indigestible plant residues. Whole grains, legumes, vegetables, and fruits in their natural unrefined state contain large amounts of fiber. This fiber is lost when flour is sifted, rice polished, or fruit made into juice. High-fiber, low-fat diets are associated with a low incidence of cardiovascular disease as well as with lowered rates of cancer of the colon, rectum, and breast. Some research epidemiologists believe that the cancer prevention associated with high-fiber diets is attributable to the relatively low amount of fat often found in such diets (rather than to the presence of fiber itself).

Further anti-cancer benefit comes from four substances called antioxidants: vitamin C, vitamin E, beta carotene, and indoles. These four antioxidants are widely present in the plant kingdom and are needed for plant survival in the plants own "hostile" environments. They therefore act as friendly co-workers along with fiber as aids in *human* survival. Antioxidants protect cells from the damage that occurs from cancer-promoting chemicals that we may take in from our food or water and also from the damaging agents called "free radicals" formed continuously as a normal process within our own bodies. Epidemiologists at the National Cancer Institute have estimated that at least 25,000 out of 100,000 deaths per year from cancers of the colon, rectum, and breast could be prevented by moderate substitutions of high-fiber vegetable foods for high-saturated-fat foods. More extensive dietary changes might provide even greater preventive benefits. Epidemiologists Dr. Richard Doll and Richard Peto of Oxford estimate as much as 80 percent of these cancers might be prevented through dietary changes.

Because we have considerably less data on the relationship between nutrition and cancer prevention than on that between nutrition and cardiovascular disease, further research is clearly needed to understand better what dietary changes might be of benefit in cancer prevention. In its 1982 publication "Diet, Nutrition and Cancer," however, the National Research Council reaffirmed that lower fat intake is associated with lower incidence of cancer, especially of the colon and breast. This publication stresses the importance of increasing the consumption of fiber-containing cereal grains, fresh fruits and vegetables and of decreasing the consumption of salt-cured foods, fat, and alcohol.

The evidence for a protective role of fiber has recently become so convincing that in 1985 the National Cancer Institute began to recommend the consumption of more low-fat, high-fiber foods. Therefore, our current knowledge strongly suggests that a return to a low-animal-fat, high-fiber diet through the use of "whole" foods such as fiber-rich fruits and vegetables and whole-grained cereals is an important step toward better nutritional health, including a lowering of the incidence of diet-related cancer.

THE PROTEIN MYTH

For generations, Americans have been taught that a healthy diet should include large amounts of protein from the "meat group" and the "dairy group"—along the lines of "the more, the better." On the contrary, most of us do *not* need all the animal protein we consume. There is no nutritional advantage in consuming much more than the minimum daily requirement of protein (about 10 percent of total calories consumed), provided that the protein is balanced and of high quality. People in many other cultures who consume a total amount of protein comparable to that consumed by Americans (about 14 percent of total calories) but whose diet is considerably lower in animal protein are just as strong and vigorous as we are. Indeed, they are probably much healthier than the average American, because their protein is derived from sources that are not high in saturated fat and cholesterol. Traditional sources of protein in the typical American diet are laden with fat. A "choice" grade of cooked, untrimmed sirloin steak, for instance, is 70 percent fat in terms of caloric value; even after trimming it is still 45 percent fat. About 70 percent of the calories in most cheeses come from butterfat. Fortunately the beef and dairy industries are now producing a larger number of low-fat products.

Outside of North America, northern Europe, Australia, and New Zealand, most people eat comparatively small quantities of meat, milk products, and eggs. A near-vegetarian diet can provide a protein level that is more than adequate. Although no single vegetable or grain supplies all the essential amino acids (the building blocks of protein) needed by humans, proper mixtures of complementary vegetables do provide all the balanced, high-quality protein that is needed in a healthy diet. Cuisines of the Middle East, the Mediterranean, Central and Latin America, and northern Africa rely heavily on such combinations (e.g., beans and rice or pastas, or beans and corn tortillas).

THE WHOLE MILK MYTH

The idea that "milk is good for you" is deeply ingrained in our culture. We were taught in school that adults need two glasses of milk a day (or the equivalent in other dairy products) and children four glasses. Numerous books and articles on nutrition provide such standard recommendations. These recommendations are sound in all respects except that nonfat milk or yogurt should be used in place of whole milk. All the protein, minerals (such as calcium), and needed vitamins are in the nonfat products. We should change our Whole Milk Myth to the Nonfat Milk Truth!

One argument from a historical or anthropologic standpoint against the need for adults to ingest large quantities of milk comes from relatively recent findings suggesting that most of the world's ethnic groups lose their ability to digest lactose (milk sugar) in early childhood. In 1974 two pediatricians, Dr. John Johnson and Dr. Norman Kretchmer, collaborated with a geographer, Dr. Frederick Simoons, in publishing a survey of critical importance to the calcium debate. Entitled "Lactose Malabsorption: Its Biology and History" (*Advances in Pediatrics*, vol. 21, 1974), the article explores the geographical, genetic, and cultural issues behind one startling fact: Between the ages of three and five, most people lose the enzyme required for the proper breakdown and absorption of lactose. Although people who cannot assimilate lactose may be able to use the protein and calcium from milk, the undigested lactose creates intestinal discomfort as it ferments in the colon; very little milk can be tolerated without causing bloating, stomach cramps, and/or diarrhea.

According to this evidence, it is primarily a few pastoral African tribes, a few ethnic groups in India, and about 80 percent of peoples of northern European ancestry that retain the critical enzyme that allows lactose absorption after the age of five. Apparently, the ability to digest lactose is the result of a genetic mutation that occurred some 10,000 years ago. In areas where people began to domesticate cattle for milk, this aberration persisted because individuals capable of taking advantage of an abundant milk supply had a selective advantage over their fellows in the struggle for survival. Dairying, however, did not spread among the indigenous populations of most areas of Asia, the Americas, the South Pacific basin, or central Africa. Some lactose nondigesters do come from cultures that have traditionally used milk. In general, such individuals can digest some forms of dairy products (e.g., natural yogurt, aged cheese, or fermented milk) in which the lactose has been largely broken down or "predigested," thus making it more easily absorbed.

As large percentages of people cannot properly digest lactose, it plainly makes no sense to promote the indiscriminate quaffing of whole milk. Even those people fortunate enough to possess the critical enzyme would do well to cut down their intake of whole-milk dairy products. Unless people limit their dairy intake to nonfat milk or low-fat cottage cheese, they consume far greater quantities of butterfat than is healthy.

Considerable interest has been generated in the issue of calcium requirements. Nonfat milk products are an excellent source of calcium, and many American women should increase their intake of calcium from such foods as one way to help prevent osteoporosis. Nonetheless, I recommend a major reduction in butterfat intake. You can obtain all the calcium you need from a varied diet that includes nonfat milk and low-fat cottage cheese (or nonfat or low-fat natural yogurt and/or fermented milk if you are a lactose non-digester) and is well represented in whole cereal grains (which contain more calcium than do refined cereals) and vegetables (such as broccoli, chard, greens, and artichokes, which are high in calcium). Avoiding soft drinks, many of which contain phosphate, is a wise precaution, because the presence of phosphate in the intestine can decrease the amount of calcium that is absorbed.

THE RICH-FOOD FIXATION

Another health hazard is created by our cultural fetish for rich foods. We tend to equate power, wealth, and status with foods that are creamy, smooth, and often white. The origin of our rich-food fixation is obscure; it may have begun in earlier eras of relative poverty when only the affluent could afford refined sugar, white flour, or cream. Meat is another symbol of affluence. Regardless of the origins of our fascination with rich foods, there is no doubt that our culture (through advertising) reinforces our desire for buttery, creamy, sauce-laden offerings. The fact that modern technology allows huge quantities of sugar and animal fat to be produced, stored, and shipped should not lead us unwittingly to consume foods that damage our cardiovascular health, promote obesity and diabetes, or induce cancer.

WHAT CAN BE DONE?

When we look at the typical American food pattern, we find a diet replete with processed foods from which many nutritionally valuable components have been removed and replaced by too much salt, too much sugar, and too many artificially hardened fats. The availability of convenient snack foods and fast-food restaurants has enticed us into eating large quantities of junk foods and eating them rapidly, often "on the run" and in an atmosphere of stress. We have received much nutritional misinformation about our true need for protein and for many years we have been surrounded by a culture that encourages us to consume far more calories, sugar, fat, and cholesterol than is healthy. A basic question becomes apparent: Since the harmful effects of the average American diet have been known for many years (the relationship of salt to high blood pressure, for instance, is "rediscovered" about every 25 years), why are steps not taken to correct the situation?

The obstacles to major dietary changes are formidable. One important constraint is scientific conservatism. It is difficult to achieve a consensus among scientists and physicians regarding the need to modify specific food hazards. Scientists and politicians hate to "tamper" with food practices that they see as firmly entrenched in the culture. The giant lobbying arms of the food industry—the processors and distributors, the fast-food franchisers and sugar refiners, the interest groups representing eggs, cheese, meat, and milk—are another powerful force for maintaining the status quo. Still, a steady assault by nutritionists, cardiovascular epidemiologists, the American Heart Association, the National Cancer Institute, and other groups is slowly overcoming these barriers. In the 1980s we are beginning to witness changes in food-buying habits, resulting from new knowledge about nutrition. There is a growing interest in natural and fiber-containing foods and a shift to lower consumption of meat and high-fat dairy products. These trends are impressive and many beneficial changes in food production and processing have already occurred. Fortunately some elements of the food industry are responding well to these new consumer demands.

Man is a highly adaptable species with a tolerance for a wide spectrum of food tastes. There is no biological factor that inhibits our ability to reshape our food preferences. In my view, people only *think* that they eat what they like; in truth they eat what they have *learned* to like. Although sweeping changes in food habits are unlikely to occur on a national scale in the forseeable future, adoption of a healthier diet can begin in your own family *now*. Such changes are not difficult provided thay are gradual.

In this chapter I will present a three-phase program for adopting an alternative food pattern. (I am indebted to Dr. William Connor for the phase concept of achieving changes in food patterns, and the American Heart Association now also advocates a phased approach.) I suggest that you allow approximately one year for each phase, although the time period can vary depending on personal preference and the ease with which you are able to bring about the desired changes. Thus, it might take some people three years to reach Phase III, others five years. Still others may prefer to stay at Phase II. By proceeding slowly, you can avoid feelings of deprivation during the change process. Try to bring about changes so subtle that neither your palate nor your attachment to particular foods suffers. Individuals with a health problem, such as a high cholesterol level or coronary artery disease, may of course elect to move much more rapidly.

Don't make yourself uncomfortable as you alter your food-related habits. Instead anticipate a new set of pleasures as you introduce yourself to new food textures and flavors. If you love to cook, all the better; the foods you eat need not be health hazards to taste good!

FOOD IDENTIFICATION

Before embarking on a change program, you need a simple method to evaluate various nutritional aspects of your current diet as well as nutritional information about the foods recommended in the alternative food pattern. What follows is a system that allows you to identify harmful, neutral, and beneficial constituents of various foods. This method focuses on monitoring the *number of times* per day or week that you consume various types of foods rather than the *amount* you consume, and it allows you to avoid complexities of weighing, measuring, and learning the exact calorie count of numerous foods. (Recording food-use frequency also facilitates switching to alternative foods, whereas cutting down on portion sizes does not.) By substituting healthy foods for "artery blockers," you retrain your palate to enjoy alternative flavors (e.g., eating strawberries with fresh lemon rather than with a smaller-than-usual amount of cream and sugar).

The chart on pages 114-115 lists foods according to their *caloric density* (which refers to the relative amount of calories found in equivalent weights of a particular food)—high, medium, or low— and also divides these foods into two broad groups: (1) those common in the typical U.S. diet (upper portion of the chart) and (2) those recommended in the alternative food pattern (lower portion of the chart). You can see from the key why the foods above the line can, when eaten too frequently, be considered unhealthy. I suggest that over the next two or three years you move *down* the chart to

CALORIC DENSITY AND SALT, SUGAR, AND SATURATED-FAT CONTENT OF COMMON FOODS

Key: SF = saturated fat; C = cholesterol; Sa = salt; Su = sugar

	High Caloric Density (HCD)	Medium Caloric Density (MCD)	Low Caloric Density (LCD)
USUAL U.S. FOOD PATTERN	Commercial baked goods and cakes made from mixes (SF, C, Sa, Su) Frankfurter (SF, C, Sa) Bacon (SF, C, Sa) Luncheon meat (SF, C, Sa) Ham, sausage (SF, C, Sa) Most regular cheeses (SF, C, Sa) Ice cream, ice milk (SF, C, Su) Creamy peanut butter (SF, Sa) Red meat (SF, C) Organ meat (SF, C) Butter (SF, C) Snack crackers (SF, Sa) Palm oil, coconut oil (SF) Hardened margarines (SF) Candy (Su) Fruit in heavy syrup (Su) Sherbet and frozen yogurt (Su) Salted nuts (Sa) Potato chips and other chips (Sa)	Buttermilk (SF, C, Sa) Egg yolk (SF, C) Whole milk (SF, C) Granolas with added salt and sugar (Sa, Su) Shellfish (C) Turkey franks (Sa) Roasting turkey injected with salt (Sa) Canned soups (Sa) Canned corn, beans, or peas (Sa) Frozen fish (Sa) Canned tuna (Sa) Biscuits, muffins, pancakes (Sa) Instant cereals (Sa) Dehydrated potatoes (Sa) All-Bran, Bran flakes, cornflakes (Sa) Soda crackers (Sa) Soft drinks (Su) *Low in fiber, but otherwise "heart healthy"* White bread, English muffins White rice Spaghetti and other pasta made from white flour Fruit juice without pulp	Bouillon (Sa) Consommé (Sa) Canned vegetable juice (Sa) Most canned garden vegetables (Sa) A few frozen vegetables (peas, succotash, lima beans) (Sa) Pickles (Sa) Sauerkraut (Sa) Melba toast (Sa) Salted popcorn (Sa)
ALTERNATIVE FOOD PATTERN	All vegetable oils (*including* olive oil) except palm and coconut Avocado Honey Mayonnaise or salad dressing Natural peanut butter (no salt) Sesame butter Sesame seeds	Breads, whole-grain Brown rice Canned fruit (no syrup) Chicken without skin Common potato and corn Egg whites Fresh fish Fresh or dried fruit Fruit juice with pulp Granolas without salt or sugar	Alfalfa sprouts and bean sprouts Artichokes Beets Broccoli Brussels sprouts Cabbage Carrots Cauliflower Celery Chard Cucumbers

Soft margarine	Legumes (beans,	Fresh vegetable juice
Sunflower seeds	lentils, peas, soy	Green beans
Unsalted nuts	beans, garbanzo	Lettuce
	beans)	Mushrooms
	Low-fat cottage cheese	Radishes
	Nonfat milk or yogurt	Spinach and other
	Puffed rice	greens
	Shredded wheat	Squash
	Spaghetti and other	Tomatoes and most
	pasta (from partial	other garden
	whole-wheat	vegetables
	varieties)	Most frozen vegetables
	Turkey	
	Yams and sweet	
	potatoes	

ALTERNATIVE FOOD PATTERN

foods low in saturated fat, cholesterol, salt, and sugar and, particularly if weight is a problem, to the *right* of the table toward foods lower in caloric density. I will not ask you to completely abandon the upper part of the chart, although over a period of time you can reduce greatly the frequency with which you consume sugary, salty, fatty, and cholesterol-laden foods.

Since fat contains nine calories per gram (compared to four calories per gram for pure carbohydrate or protein), fatty foods (sausage, frankfurters, red meat, cheese, nuts, avocados, mayonnaise, and table spreads) are listed as high caloric density (HCD). Meats lower in fat content (poultry or fish) are medium caloric density. Cereals (wheat, corn, and rice), root vegetables (potatoes), and legumes (beans, peas, and lentils), all of which contain relatively large amounts of water, fiber, and starchy carbohydrates, are also classified as medium caloric density (MCD). Common garden vegetables or vegetable juices are the major constituents of the low-caloric-density (LCD) list, primarily because of their relatively high water content and secondarily because of their fiber content. Noncaloric constituents, water and fiber, not only dilute the calories of vaious foods, but also slow down our caloric intake. These satiate the appetite partially because of their bulk and partially because the relatively longer time it takes to eat them allows the appetite center in the brain to register that the blood sugar level has risen and that we have satisfied our true hunger.

To gain further knowledge of food constituents and nutritional values of various foods, you may wish to read further (see Reader's Guide for suggestions). However, directing your attention to the number of times a day that you eat foods high in sugar, salt, saturated fat, and cholesterol will provide you with a basic, manageable framework for attaining a healthy food pattern.

ONE: IDENTIFYING YOUR FOOD-PATTERN PROBLEMS

The first step in a program to lower your food-related chronic disease risk is to gauge your current risk level by referring to the Simplified Self-Scoring Test of Chronic Disease Risk (see pages 38-39). The average American adult has the following score:

Risk Factor 2 (Body Weight):	3 points
Risk Factor 3 (Salt Intake or Blood Pressure):	2 points
Risk Factor 4 (Saturated-Fat and Cholesterol Intake or Blood Cholesterol Level):	3 points
Total	8 points

The sum of these three food-related risk factors is about 60 percent of the average American's total chronic-disease-risk score (13 points). Food-related cardiovascular risk can easily be reduced, over a period of two to three years, to the zero- or one-point level for each of these three categories. All but a very small minority of readers will find room for needed changes in food habits. Some of you, for instance, will already be at your ideal weight. A few of you may have upper-level blood pressure readings of less than 110 millimeters, and a few others may also have blood cholesterol levels of less than 150 mg./dl. The likelihood, however, of your having *zero* or one risk point in *all three* food-related cardiovascular risk areas is extremely slight.

Even people who currently have a low food-related cardiovascular risk score can benefit from moving toward the alternative food patttern set forth here. First, it is a useful *preventive* measure since, given the same dietary intake, body weight, blood pressure, and blood cholesterol generally increase almost 1 percent per year from ages 25 to 50; second, it is more natural, more flavorful, and less expensive; and third, it conserves food and energy resources because vegetable foods are lower on the food chain than are animal foods and are more abundant and energy efficient in their production. (See Frances Moore Lappé's *Diet for a Small Planet* for an excellent description of the economics of our current agricultural practices and the food-chain concept.)

TWO: BUILDING COMMITMENT

Although you may now realize intellectually that changing your food habits would be sensible, you may still have strongly entrenched beliefs that could be significant barriers to change. Examine your attitudes. What obstacles do you encounter when you contemplate making changes in your food pattern? Take note of random thoughts that cast light on your willingness to proceed. Make a list of your belief barriers and then devise a list of rational counterarguments. Practice refuting your belief barriers with these counterarguments a few times a day for several weeks. Your list might look like the following:

ATTITUDES THAT INHIBIT OR FACILITATE SUCCESS IN ADOPTING AN ALTERNATIVE FOOD PATTERN

Belief Barriers	Effective Counterarguments
1. I don't want to give up all the foods I enjoy. Who wants to suffer?	1. Food preferences are learned. I don't have to give up all my favorite foods. I can learn to enjoy new flavors. It's worth trying.
2. Medical scientists don't all agree about the relationship between nutrition, heart disease, and cancer.	2. There is strong evidence that food patterns have a significant bearing on cardiovascular health and cancer. I'd rather be safe than wait for everything to be "proven" conclusively.
3. I'm afraid that changing my food pattern would be too difficult.	3. Gradual changes using the simplified methods described in this book are manageable. The family can make this a cooperative effort.
4. I'm concerned that changing to an alternative food pattern will be more expensive.	4. Eating lower on the food chain is *less* expensive. We can cut our meat bills in half.
5. My family and I are healthy.	5. We aren't sick that often, but our food pattern doesn't sound as healthy as I once thought it was. Lowering our salt, sugar, and saturated-fat intake, while increasing our fiber intake, will be far healthier in the long run for the entire family.

6. Changing to the alternative food pattern makes me feel that I am rejecting the life-style my family has always enjoyed.

6. It's important to make changes when they are warranted by new knowledge. We can make changes gradually so that everyone becomes comfortable with them.

7. In the long run we all die anyway, so why bother?

7. My example can help the rest of my family change their diet and improve their health. I'm not a defeatist about the possibility and desirability of change. It will be worth the effort. Why needlessly risk preventable cancer and heart disease?

8. (fill in) _____

8. (fill in) _____

9. (fill in) _____

9. (fill in) _____

Your motivation to continue increases as you overcome your belief barriers. Augment your confidence and commitment by involving family members and/or friends in your program.

THREE: DEVELOPING AWARENESS OF FOOD INTAKE PATTERNS

As you prepare for your change effort, estimate how frequently you consume foods that contain saturated fat, cholesterol, sugar, and salt. Also determine how many high-caloric-density foods you eat daily. The sample menu (typical of current U.S. food patterns) on page 119 demonstrates the scoring system that helps you evaluate your current food intake.

Although this system emphasizes *how often* you consume particular types of foods rather than *how much* you consume, if a portion is unusually large (e.g., more than six ounces of meat) allow two negative points for each relevant category instead of one. To gain a more accurate appraisal of your current food pattern as well as practice in classifying foods, record your own menus for a week or two. Remember that packaged commercial foods often contain high levels of salt, sugar, and hydrogenated oils (saturated fat).

Awareness of food patterns extends to issues beyond the frequency with which you consume various kinds of food. Food buying and storage habits, eating speed, eating location, and meal and snacking frequency are aspects of your food pattern that will be discussed in Chapter 7 (Weight Control). If you have weight problems, you will want to use Chapters 6 and 7 in conjunction with one another.

Another aspect of your eating habits that deserves attention is the spacing of meals. People who skip breakfast or lunch are apt to eat

---

SAMPLE MENU—USUAL U.S. FOOD PATTERN

Breakfast	Points	Lunch	Points
1 cup coffee with 2 teaspoons		Sandwich, 2 slices white	
of sugar (Su) (HCD)	= –2	bread with salami (SF) (C)	
Orange juice		(Sa) (HCD) and	= –4
Bacon – 2 slices (SF) (C) (Sa)		cheese (SF) (C) (Sa) (HCD)	= –4
(HCD)	= –4	1 piece of cake (SF) (Su) (Sa)	
Toast – 2 slices with margarine		(HCD)	= –4
(SF) (HCD)	= –2	2 pickles (Sa)	= –1
and jam (Su) (HCD)	= –2		–13
	–10		

		Dinner	
Snacks		1 glass whole milk (SF) (C)	= –2
Cola drink (Su)	= –1	2 slices white bread with hard	
3 cookies (SF) (Su) (Sa)		margarine (SF) (HCD)	= –2
(HCD)	= –4	Meat loaf (SF) (C) (HCD)	= –3
Salted peanuts (Sa) (HCD)	= –2	Mashed potatoes with salt	= –1
Sweet roll (SF) (Su) (Sa)		(Sa) and hard margarine	
(HCD)	= –4	(SF) (HCD)	= –2
	–11	Frozen peas (Sa)	= –1
		Ice Cream (Su) (SF) (C)	
Key		(HCD)	= –4
Sugar = (Su)			–15
Salt = (Sa)			

Key
Sugar = (Su)
Salt = (Sa)
Saturated Fat = (SF)
Cholesterol = (C)
High-Caloric-Density
 Food = (HCD)

Total Score = –49 points. U.S. average range = –40 to –50 points

Score for frequency of use:

Sugar	= –7	Saturated fat	= –12	High-caloric-	
Salt	= –10	Cholesterol	= –6	density	= –14

Scoring system: Allow one negative point for each category in which a portion of food is high in (1) sugar, (2) salt, (3) saturated fat, (4) cholesterol, and/or (5) caloric density. (Consider 2 teaspoons of sugar as one portion, 2 slices of bread or 3 cookies as one portion, and 2 teaspoons of butter, margarine, or table spread as one portion.)

more heavily at the evening meal than they otherwise would. Large evening meals or late evening snacks often result in general lassitude or insomnia stemming from incomplete digestion. Large noon meals are often followed by lowered mental alertness and sometimes by weakness, headaches, or hand tremors. Some of these symptoms are attributable to a mild form of hypoglycemia (low blood sugar) that occurs after a high influx of calories into the bloodstream. As the calories are absorbed, the blood-sugar level increases markedly, which in turn triggers the production of insulin as the body attempts to bring the blood-sugar level back into balance. The higher-than-normal insulin level then abruptly lowers the blood-sugar level, resulting in hypoglycemia. Such problems can be minimized by proper meal spacing, avoidance of too many sugary HCD foods, and increased levels of physical activity (which seem to decrease broad swings in blood-sugar levels).

FOUR: DEVELOPING AN ACTION PLAN FOR CHANGE

After gaining an awareness of the negative aspects of your current eating pattern, you are ready to devise an action plan to move gradually toward an alternative food pattern. The action plan for this effort has three phases, as mentioned earlier, each of which is about one year in duration. Major changes in life-style are often needed to change food habits. It will take patience and persistence to retrain your palate to enjoy new foods and to adjust to new recipes that are compatible with the alternative food pattern. The point is to bring about permanent changes—not temporary ones.

Within a few years you can comfortably adjust to a diet containing one-quarter or less of the average U.S. intake of saturated fat, cholesterol, refined sugar, salt, and high-caloric-density "convenience" foods. By adopting the alternative food pattern recommended here, you will double your intake of high-fiber, complex-carbohydrate foods, such as whole-grained cereal products, legumes, and common garden vegetables. This more than doubles your protein intake from vegetable sources and, when combined with an exercise program, provides an effective way to shed unwanted pounds and keep them off.

As of 1978, a total of 16 national and international advisory bodies (including the American Heart Association, the American Cancer Society, the National Academy of Sciences, and the Departments of Health of Great Britain, Sweden, and Norway) had recommended nutritional and body-weight goals for all adults that approximate Phase I of this program. The American Heart Association's 1986 diet recommendations have become more advanced and are now close to the Phase II level. I believe that adopting the food pattern of Phase III is even more desirable from the standpoint of preventing diet-related cancer and cardiovascular disease. Nonetheless, if you are more comfortable at Phase I or II, these will provide considerable benefit. If you have a strong family history of coronary disease or an inborn tendency to a high cholesterol level, then a Phase III approach is needed and your physician may need to add cholesterol-lowering drugs as well.

PHASE I

General Instructions. Phase I is the initial transition from the average American diet to the alternative food pattern; this is a distinctly non-threatening phase. In Phase I you retain most of your present food habits but substitute alternatives for foods highest in salt, sugar, saturated fat, and cholesterol. Your total daily negative point score (calculated as in the sample menu, page 119) should decrease by about one-third (e.g., from the U.S. average range of minus 40 to minus 50 to a range of minus 25 to minus 35 a day).

The changes to be made in Phase I are listed below, followed by time schedule, and instructions for carrying out the changes.

PHASE I CHANGES

A. Saturated-Fat and Cholesterol Control
  1. Reduce weekly servings of whole milk, cheese (other than low-fat cottage cheese), fatty meats (beef, lamb, bacon, spareribs, sausage, and luncheon meats), and ice cream by one-half (e.g., from the U.S. average of 24 servings a week to about a combined total of 12 per week). Substitute complex-carbohydrate foods and foods such as fish and poultry in their place. (Do not eat chicken skin.)
  2. Change from ice cream to ice milk and from whole milk to nonfat milk. (Infants should preferably be breast-fed. If infants are formula-fed, use the "natural" low-sodium varieties that have recently become available. If they are given cow's milk, use whole milk only up to the age of two years.)
  3. Reduce meat fat by trimming and by broiling or roasting instead of frying.
  4. Eliminate intake of organ meats such as liver, sweetbreads, and brains.

5. Change from butter or hard margarine (made with hydrogenated oil) to soft tub margarine (made with unhydrogenated oil).
6. Change from lard or shortening to unhydrogenated vegetable oil, including olive oil if desired. (Although some nutritonists recommend use of the most highly polyunsaturated oils, I feel that any type of vegetable oil other than palm or coconut oil [the only saturated fats that are liquid at room temperature] is acceptable. Healthy cultures have used olive oil, a mono-unsaturated oil, successfully for thousands of years.) Avoid use of large amounts of vegetable oils, as you want to lower your total fat intake in Phase I from the current U.S. average of 40 percent to about 30 percent of total calories consumed. Furthermore, large amounts of polyunsaturated fats may contribute to cancer risk.
7. Reduce consumption of egg yolks to no more than four a week. Use egg whites liberally.
8. Change from creamy peanut butter made with hydrogenated fat to natural peanut butter made without hydrogenated fat.
9. Reduce consumption of fast foods, processed and convenience foods, commercial baked goods, and the like.

B. Sugar Control
1. Reduce consumption of soft drinks by half. Limit intake to two or three a week. (U.S. average is five 12-ounce cans or bottles a week.)
2. Gradually eliminate the use of sugar in coffee or tea and on fruit. (Saccharin use is discouraged, not only because of its possible role as a carcinogen but also because of the importance of retraining your palate to lowered sweetness levels.)
3. Switch from heavy to light syrup in canned fruits.
4. Substitute fruit for pastry, cake, pie, or other sweets in one-third of all desserts.

C. Salt and Caffeine Control
1. Eliminate, except for rare use, high-salt items such as bacon, ham, sausage, frankfurters, luncheon meats, salted nuts, sauerkraut, pickles, canned soups, canned vegetables, potato chips, and other salted snack foods.
2. Switch from regular table salt to a light salt (one-half sodium chloride, one-half potassium chloride).

3. Gradually decrease salt use in cooking to about one-third previous levels; simultaneously decrease, and eventually eliminate, salt use at the table.
4. Explore the use of other flavors in your cooking—spices, herbs, lemon, wine, vinegar, etc.
5. Limit intake of caffeinated drinks (coffee, tea, cola, etc.) to four cups a day. Try decaffeinated alternatives and herb teas.

D. Complex-Carbohydrate and Fiber Control
1. Increase intake of complex-carbohydrate foods—including legumes (e.g., beans, peas, lentils), starchy root vegetables such as the potato, as well as other vegetables and fruits—as a partial or full caloric replacement (depending on weight-control needs) for reduced intake of sugar and fatty animal foods.
2. Gradually introduce whole-grained cereals into your food plan (e.g., whole-wheat bread and flour, bulgur, couscous, cracked wheat, rolled oats, rye, brown rice, etc.).
3. Increase intake of whole fruits (fruit juices lack much of the fiber contained in whole fruits).
4. Increase intake of whole vegetables (vegetable juices lack much of the fiber contained in whole vegetables and often contain significant amounts of added salt).

E. High-Caloric-Density Food Control
1. Reduce intake of HCD foods by one-third (e.g., from average U.S. number of 15 portions per day to about 10 per day). By doing this, you will also reduce your intake of salt, sugar, and saturated fat.
2. Partially or fully replace such foods with complex carbohydrates (depending on weight-control goals).

F. Alcohol Control
1. Because alcohol may add to weight-control problems and may displace valuable nutrients, limit alcohol consumption so that no more than 5 percent of your total calorie intake is derived from alcohol, e.g., approximately one bottle of beer (12 oz.) or two glasses of wine (6 oz.) or one cocktail (1½ oz. liquor) per day.

Before you launch your Phase I efforts, gather some cookbooks that will help make the transition to a healthier eating pattern more pleasurable. Three books that suggest many excellent recipes are *Jane Brody's Good Food Book*, *Diet for a Small Planet* by Frances Moore Lappé, and *Recipes for a Small Planet* by Ellen Buchman Ewald. The last 15 years have seen the publication of a large number of excellent recipe books that can be used to implement the suggestions we are making in this chapter. They introduce you in a pleasant and often exciting way to diets lower in animal fat and higher in carbohydrates, such as those exemplified by Mediterranean and Middle Eastern cuisines. Look for this type of book in your bookstore. Some suggestions are given in the Reader's Guide at the end of this book. I am not suggesting that you need plunge immediately into a sea of alien new dishes, but even in the early stages of your palate's re-education it is helpful to expose yourself to interesting recipes for foods low in sugar, salt, saturated fat, and cholesterol. Cutting down on salt is made easier by learning to flavor your foods with an expanded range of herbs, spices, and condiments (e.g., see the herb and spice sections of *The Joy of Cooking* by Irma Rombauer and Marion Becker).

Clearly, your family or eating partners should share in your venture since separate meal preparation is not likely to be maintained. If your family does not fully participate in pursuing the health themes of this book, approach the food-pattern changes from the standpoint of encouraging your family to join you in discovering more interesting and more flavorful foods. As a financial incentive, monitor your food bills before and after embarking on Phase I to discover how much money you save.

If you are to achieve lasting changes in your diet, I suggest that you adopt a clear-cut structure for achieving these goals. Don't try to make all the changes at once. Rather, concentrate on one or two problem areas at a time (e.g., for two or three months each). Assuming that you allow yourself a full year to achieve Phase I, you will have a period of several months to work on maintaining the changes you have brought about (further adjusting to your new way of eating) before you embark on Phase II.

Figure 6-2 depicts a typical 12-month sequence for achieving the Phase I changes. This blueprint provides a schematic way of proceeding. Some people may prefer a longer change period, others a shorter one. Be guided by your own ability to achieve the changes comfortably. In this blueprint there is one three-month block (A) and two two-month blocks (B and C). Each block is ushered in with an extra push and, once the changes are attained, a leisurely maintenance effort continues throughout the rest of Phase I.

The sequence of working to achieve fat and sugar control (Block A), then salt and caffeine control (Block B), and finally high-caloric-density food and alcohol control (Block C) is optimal—unless a person has blood pressure upper-level readings of 150 or higher, in which case salt control is the most pressing need and Block B offers a prompt way to help lower blood pressure. Block A is the area that, generally speaking, requires the greatest amount of effort to bring about lasting changes. Changes made in Block A (substitution of alternative foods for foods high in saturated fat or sugar) help facilitate subsequent changes in Blocks B and C, since many high-fat and high-sugar foods are also high in salt and/or caloric density.

Embarking on Phase I

Let me now discuss a sample Phase I program (I will assume that you are following the A, B, C sequence). As you begin, I suggest that you resolve to make specific substitutions for various high-fat and high-sugar foods that you eat regularly. Refer to the chart on pages 114 and 115. The foods you will be cutting down on will come from the HCD section of the "Usual U.S. Food Pattern" (most red meats and whole-milk dairy products are in this section). Now review the

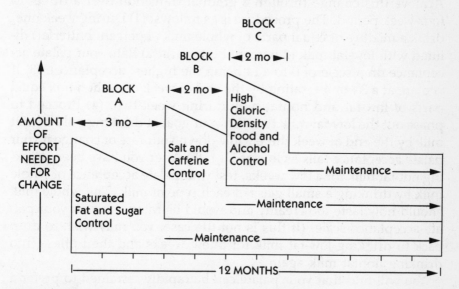

Figure 6-2: Blueprint for Adoption of Alternative Food Pattern

list of foods in the "Alternative Food Pattern." You will be choosing substitutes from this list, most of which will probably come from the MCD section (whole-grained cereals, poultry, fish, fruits, legumes, and root vegetables). You will also use some HCD alternates (soft margarine, unsalted peanut butter, nuts, avocados, etc.) and many LCD alternates (most common garden vegetables).

Any change plan should be based on observations of your usual eating pattern as revealed in a two-week record of your food intake. Your change plan should also include a palate satisfaction rating to gauge whether or not you have successfully adjusted to new foods and flavors. Build your program on small incremental changes. Do not proceed until you have adjusted comfortably to current alterations in your regular eating pattern. Devise alterations that allow you to *enjoy* your new eating pattern. For instance, during Block A, it is better to season your new foods so that you like them, even if that involves initially leaving your salt and sugar intakes at a higher level; once you adjust to new foods and flavors, you can then taper, and eventually phase out, your use of salt at the table during Block B of Phase I and taper your sugar use during Block C.

An early change that is readily achieved is to substitute nonfat milk for whole milk. This has the twin virtues of being simple and of demonstrating the palate's adaptability to new flavors and textures. Achieve this change through a gradual transition over a three- to four-week period. The procedure is as follows: (1) During week one, drink a mixture of equal parts of whole milk (4 percent butterfat) diluted with low-fat milk (2 percent butterfat). (2) Rate your palate acceptance on a scale of 0 to 4 (4 being the highest acceptance). (3) If you are at a 3+ or 4+ rating by the end of week one, then mix equal parts of low-fat and nonfat milk during week two. (4) Proceed to phase out the low-fat milk to reach your goal of drinking only nonfat milk by the end of week three (slow down your rate of change if your palate acceptance falls as low as 2+). (5) After you have been drinking nonfat milk for a few weeks, test your palate acceptance of whole milk by drinking a small glass of each type of milk. The whole milk should now taste too creamy and would be rated *lower* on your palate-acceptance scale. (If this is not the case, you may wish to drop back to drinking low-fat milk for a few weeks and then phase into drinking nonfat milk again.)

You will find that your palate can be rapidly retrained to prefer a new flavor. Here are some other changes that can be accomplished without much difficulty: (1) In home cooking, use liquid vegetable oils rather than lard or shortening (which are predominately saturated fat). (2) Change from butter or hard, hydrogenated margarine to soft, unhydrogenated margarine. If you find it difficult to give up butter, experiment with new flavors and textures that will offset the loss of the butter flavor. (3) Change from creamy or cheese-based salad dressings to vinegar-and-oil based dressings or even to commercial salad dressings and/or mayonnaise (which may contain small amounts of egg yolk but are nonetheless a considerable improvement over creamy or cheese-based varieties).

For the first few weeks, concentrate on making these relatively simple changes. Once you are confident that your palate accepts these substitutes, you are ready to undertake more complex changes. I suggest that you focus on particular meals since eating habits are usually quite specific for breakfast, lunch, dinner, and snacks. For example, your next step could be to alter the foods you eat for breakfast. This is generally the easiest meal to change since in most households breakfast choices can be individualized. The sample self-contract that follows demonstrates how you might proceed:

PHASE I BLOCK A: SELF-CONTRACT FOR BREAKFAST CHANGES

I have decided to substitute foods from the alternative food pattern for a number of my usual breakfast foods as my next two-week goal. My helper will be _____.

On four mornings a week I will substitute the following alternates for my usual breakfast of bacon and eggs: (1) shredded wheat in nonfat milk with sliced bananas and honey; (2) rye or whole-wheat toast spread with peanut butter and chopped dates or raisins; (3) broiled toasted English muffins with soft margarine, sliced tomato, and sliced low-fat mozzarella cheese; (4) scrambled egg substitute and rye or whole-wheat toast with soft margarine.

My responsibilities are (1) to purchase the alternative foods and prepare them, (2) to record the number of times I eat alternative foods and the palate satisfaction I achieve (on a scale of 0 to 4), (3) to use extra salt or honey as needed to flavor foods, (4) to tape this contract on the refrigerator door as a reminder.

My helper's responsibilities are (1) to remind me to eat these alternatives instead of my usual breakfast foods, (2) to participate in and support my efforts to change our usual breakfast patterns.

Our joint responsibility is to evaluate the results of the program weekly and to make revisions as needed.

Date: _____   Signed: _____
Review Date: _____   Helper: _____

If you intend to bring about the Phase I fat-control and sugar-control changes in three months, try to achieve your breakfast alterations in about two weeks. Allot a similar time period for achieving lunch, dinner, snack, and eating-out changes. If two-week intervals rush you too much, slow down. Allow yourself to adjust to one group of changes before going on to the next. In addition to the books previously mentioned, the following contain recipes that will furnish ideas for your Phase I meals and snacks: *The American Heart Association Cookbook* and *The New American Diet* by Sonja and William Connor.

Here are a few suggestions for Phase I lunches and dinners low in saturated fat and sugar: turkey or chicken sandwiches on whole-wheat bread (in place of roast beef or ham), fruit (instead of pastry), and nonfat milk (in place of whole milk); or veal, fish, or poultry (in place of beef or liver), rice or baked potatoes (in place of french fries); ice milk (in place of ice cream); and canned fruit in light (rather than heavy) syrup.

If you have trouble giving up particular foods, I suggest that you practice a Food Substitution Drill. Some people, for example, may have trouble reducing their saturated-fat intake because of cravings for particular fatty-food favorites. You may accept intellectually that it would be wise to begin replacing some of your high-fat foods with less fatty alternatives such as fish, poultry, veal, or young beef, yet you may still crave a steak, hamburger, spareribs, or the like. Using your mental imagery skills, carry out the following drill to facilitate this change. Before you begin, collect a glass of fat drippings released during the cooking of one of your favorite fatty meats (such as spareribs, bacon, hamburger, or steak) and place the glass in the refrigerator for a few hours. Then inspect the hardened fat and remove some of it in a spoon. Feel its texture. You are now ready to proceed.

FOOD SUBSTITUTION DRILL

1. Sit or lie down comfortably in a quiet room.
2. Achieve a state of partial deep muscle relaxation and mental relaxation.
3. Think of your favorite fatty meat, prepared in its usual fashion. Conjure the aroma and appearance so that you desire this food.

4. Next, think of the appearance and texture of the hardened fat drippings from this food.

5. Imagine this saturated fat as a thick sludge flowing through your arteries and slowly closing them off.

6. Couple the image of the fatty food with that of the greasy sludge until your desire for this food lessens.

7. Next, imagine a less fatty alternative food (e.g., roast turkey) complete with seasonings, etc., that make the thoughts of this food pleasant.

8. Couple the image of this food with an image of arteries that are clean and free of fatty deposits.

9. End the drill by thinking of a pleasant mental image (e.g., an image of yourself looking healthy and vital, a blue sky, a peaceful mountain lake, etc.).

This type of Food Substitution Drill can be applied to any food you wish. As you retrain your palate to enjoy alternative foods, you will have less need for the drill.

Let us suppose that after three months you have achieved the targeted changes for saturated-fat and sugar control. I suggest that for the next two months (Block B) you concentrate on cutting your current salt intake to about six grams per day (one-half the U.S. average). Also in Block B, limit your intake of caffeinated beverages (caffeine raises blood pressure) to four cups a day. You will have already achieved some salt reduction as a result of your Block A activities since many high-fat foods are also salty. You can achieve further reduction by (1) substituting alternative foods that are low in salt in place of highly salted items, (2) switching to a light salt (one-half sodium chloride, one-half potassium chloride), and (3) reducing the amount of salt used in cooking and reducing, and later eliminating, salt used at the table.

Common high-salt items include salted and/or smoked meats such as bacon, ham, sausage, frankfurters, luncheon meats. Canned soups, canned vegetables, salted nuts, potato chips, pickles, canned tuna, and pickled herring are also high in salt. Many commercial granola mixtures contain considerable amounts of salt and sugar. Frozen peas, frozen fish, buttermilk, most cheeses (except for low-fat cottage cheese), and certain commercial breakfast cereals (All-Bran and cornflakes) are quite high in added salt, whereas others (shredded wheat) are not.

Another hidden hazard is water that has been softened by a process that replaces calcium with sodium. Avoid using artificially softened water as a source of drinking or cooking water. Various antacids are very high in sodium (your druggist or physician can advise you on the few antacids that are low in sodium). Vitamin C tablets are sometimes sold in the form of sodium ascorbate, the sodium salt of ascorbic acid. It is ironic that a person may seek health "salvation" in large doses of this vitamin only to incur a rise in blood pressure!

The chart on pages 114 and 115 will help you find substitutions for some of the salty foods that you eat regularly. Create short-term self-contracts that specify your plans. For example, you might substitute unsalted crackers for salted crackers; bean sprouts for pickles in sandwiches; pork for ham; fresh vegetables for canned vegetables; lean beef, turkey, chicken, or fish for sausage, frankfurters, or luncheon meats (avoid pre-salted varieties of sliced turkey).

Practice a few substitutions over a one- or two-week period. If you are tempted by a specific food, use a Food Substitution Drill in which you associate a salty food with feeling tense and "hot under the collar" as your blood pressure rises, and a non-salty food with feeling relaxed and calm as your blood pressure decreases.

Over a two-month period, you can dramatically reduce your palate's sensitivity to salt. At the end of Block B, check your progress by drinking canned tomato or vegetable juice or eating a canned soup. If the soup or vegetable juice now tastes too salty, you have succeeded in lowering your salt threshold. (If you have not achieved sufficient progress, extend this salt-control effort until you have brought about the desired changes.)

By the end of Block B you will have mastered the main elements of Phase I. By reducing your intake of high-fat and high-sugar foods you have automatically switched to a diet lower in caloric density. You have also reduced your salt and caffeine intakes.

In Block C you focus your efforts on further reducing your HCD food intake as you maintain your changes already achieved in Blocks A and B. As you begin your Block C program, record for a one-week period the number of HCD foods you consume daily. This will let you know what changes you need to make. Say that you currently eat about 13 HCD foods per day. Devise a two-month plan in which you reduce this to ten HCD foods a day. Achieve this goal through the use of one- or two-week self-contracts that focus on substituting non-HCD foods for problem foods. For example, you may decide to concentrate first on breakfast, then on lunch, dinner, and finally snacks. If you want to lose weight (or keep pounds off), coordinate Block C with the weight control program suggested in Chapter 7 (e.g., special methods to help you control HCD-food intake, suppress eating urges, etc.). Mastering the techniques recommended in Chapter 7 will fortify your Block C efforts.

Recall that alcohol control is part of Block C and that one bottle of beer, two glasses of wine, or one cocktail generally represent the upper range of alcohol intake (limiting calories derived from alcohol to less than 5 percent of total calories). Achieve alcohol control by using the same methods you have applied to other change efforts. Identify and alter your belief barriers about lowering your alcohol intake, commit yourself to change, observe and record your drinking patterns, and devise and implement a plan of action. Urge-suppression methods such as deep muscle relaxation and physical exercise are often very helpful—particularly if you use alcohol to help relieve emotional tension. One simple step is to limit alcohol intake to beer or wine at meals, in place of before- or after-dinner drinks.

Evaluation: Phase I

Evaluate your progress throughout the first seven months of your Phase I action Plan (e.g., at the end of each one- or two-week self-contract, at the end of each block, etc.). This enables you to determine when you are ready to proceed and when you need to return to an earlier stage of identifying problems, building commitment, or increasing awareness. Again, the key to making lasting changes is to reshape your habits so that you enjoy the changes you have made. If you are not yet comfortable, determine where your problems lie—for instance, in unimaginative recipes or overperfectionist goals—and alter your program accordingly.

Maintenance: Phase I

The remaining months of Phase I allow you to consolidate your gains and work on special problems. As you look back at the Phase I changes set forth on pages 121-123, locate areas that need further attention. This might mean making systematic efforts to increase your fiber intake or to further reduce your alcohol or fatty-food intake. If you are working on a weight-control program in conjunction with your food-pattern changes, this period allows you to focus on specific ways to lose weight. Also improve your skills as a label reader and learn more about nutrition and health (see the Reader's Guide).

Reward yourself amply during this period. For instance, continue to improve the quality of the flavors you experience. Explore new foods and recipes to help you edge away from flavors achieved with salt, cream, butter, and egg yolk toward flavors achieved with herbs, spices, lemon, tomato, onion, garlic, olive oil, chili, wine, and vinegar. In addition to reaping the intrinsic pleasures of eating flavorful foods, build other forms of reward into your program. (For instance, your self-contracts could include provisions for engaging in a pleasurable activity or making a desired purchase contingent upon reaching one of your goals.)

During this time, you will gain experience in coping with special problems involving trips, parties, guests, and eating out. You can learn how to avoid having your progress sabotaged by obstacles that you encounter in your daily routine. Most restaurants have sandwiches, salads, and a variety of veal, fish, or poultry dishes that fit into a Phase I diet. (Through repeated requests you might even influence a few restaurants to make margarine and nonfat milk available.) At parties avoid overindulging in snacks and hors d'oeuvres that don't fit your new food pattern. An Instant Relaxation and Urge Suppression Drill can help steer you away from salted chips and cheese dip toward fresh vegetables or a glass of wine.

If you find yourself backsliding, repeat earlier steps that help you deal with a particular difficulty: identify the problem, build commitment, increase awareness, and finally, build a new action plan. One way of handling a craving for a particular food, for instance, is to eat the food two or three times a day for three to four days or until you have had more of it than you truly want. This heavy reexposure can sometimes rid you of "nostalgia" more effectively than can an intellectual argument. Another alternative is to use a Food Substitution Drill to suppress your craving.

When you have become comfortable with the changes you have made and with your ability to maintain them, you are ready to move on to the next stage of the alternative food pattern. I will describe both Phase II and Phase III in an abbreviated fashion in the next two sections because the methods used to bring about these changes are essentially the same as those used in Phase I.

PHASE II

General Instructions. A year or so after embarking on Phase I (or when you feel you are ready to begin Phase II), refer to the Simplified Self-Scoring Test of Chronic Disease Risk (pages 38-39). By the end of

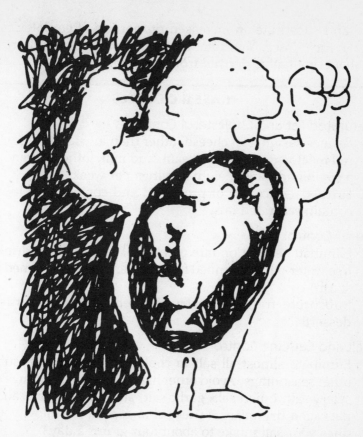

Phase I, you will have lowered your cardiovascular risk score in all three food-related areas (body weight, cholesterol level, and blood pressure level). You will have reduced your intake of red meats, whole milk and whole-milk cheeses, eggs (with yolks), and other high-saturated-fat foods to about 12 servings per week, reduced your salt intake to about six grams a day, and reduced your intake of HCD foods to about ten per day. These changes should have allowed you to lose one-third or more of your excess weight (if you were overweight).

Phase II is designed to be a year-long project for you and your family. It is a time for more radical experimentation. Become better acquainted with the foods of other cultures. Mediterranean, Mexican, Indian, and Middle Eastern cuisines, for instance, offer a multitude of healthy and delicious recipes that fit into the alternative food pattern. Phase II allows you to develop more meatless meals, or meals in which meat or cheese is used as a condiment rather than as a main component. In Phase II you further reduce the harmful dietary elements (salt, sugar, saturated fat, cholesterol, and high-caloric-density foods) and substitute an increased proportion of complex carbohydrates in their place. Your total protein intake does not decrease but now about one-half is derived from vegetable sources.

PHASE II CHANGES

A. Saturated-Fat and Cholesterol Control
1. Reduce servings of cheese (other than low-fat cottage cheese), red meat, egg yolks, ice cream, and milk (other than nonfat) to a combined total of eight servings per week.
2. Further reduce use of processed and convenience foods that contain saturated fats.

B. Sugar Control
1. Eliminate, except on rare occasions, intake of soft drinks.
2. Use water-packed canned fruit (rather than fruit canned in light syrup).
3. Substitute fruit for pastry, pie, etc., for two-thirds of all desserts.

C. Salt and Caffeine Control
1. Eliminate almost all salt in cooking of vegetables; substitute other seasonings. Avoid other high-sodium seasonings such as celery salt, onion salt, garlic salt, steak sauce, soy sauce, and packaged dry mixes. (These changes should allow you to reduce your salt intake to about four grams a day.)
2. Develop a list of no-salt-added alternatives to some of your usual foods (e.g., peanut butter, mayonnaise, catsup, and canned vegetables come in no-salt or low-salt varieties). Fresh fruits and vegetables are naturally low in salt and should be your primary substitutes.
3. Maintain intake of caffeinated beverages at no more than four cups a day. (Continue to use decaffeinated alternatives and herb teas.)

D. Complex-Carbohydrate and Fiber Control
1. Increase intake of whole-grained breads, cereals, fruits, and whole vegetables to at least five servings per day.
2. About one-half of fruit juices should contain pulp (e.g., whole citrus juice, unfiltered apple juice, etc.).

E. High-Caloric-Density Food Control
1. Further reduce intake of HCD foods to seven per day.

2. If you are working on a weight-control program (see Chapter 7), plan to reduce your remaining excess weight by one-half.

F. Alcohol Control
1. Maintain your alcohol consumption at no more than 5 percent of your total caloric intake, as in Phase I.

Before you start to make your Phase II changes, see whether or not you have any significant belief barriers about the need to make these changes or your ability to do so. When you have located and surmounted your residual belief barriers, you can make a firm commitment to proceed. Write a self-contract that involves your family or eating partners in achieving the Phase II changes.

Continue to increase your awareness of your progress by periodically testing your salt and sugar taste thresholds. For instance, does commercial cake icing seem too sweet? If you are a bit offended by the overpowering amount of sugar so often found in "improved" foods, you are making progress. Similarly, do salted nuts, ham, and bacon taste too salty?

In Phase II (and Phase III) you will be able to switch to a food-scoring method that allows you to rate foods simply as negative, neutral, or positive. As you work to bring about specific changes in Blocks A, B, and C of Phase II, record your intake of foods in the particular food categories that apply. The food-scoring method works as follows:

SIMPLIFIED FOOD-SCORING SYSTEM

1. Foods in the "Usual U.S. Food Pattern" (above the midline in the chart on pages 114-115):

Score

a. Any food with saturated fat, cholesterol, sugar, and/or salt. = −1

b. Fruit juice without pulp, white rice, foods made from white flour (foods identified as "low in fiber but otherwise 'heart healthy'"). = 0

2. Foods in the "Alternative Food Pattern" (below the midline in the chart on page 114-115):

a. Foods with fiber (any whole-grained cereal, any whole vegetable, fruit, nuts, or seeds) without saturated fats, cholesterol, sugar, and/or salt. = +1

b. Egg white, chicken without skin, turkey, fish (preferably fresh, not salted in processing).   = +1
Scores are given for an average portion size (e.g., 20 raisins = +1; 1
whole egg = -1; 2 slices whole-wheat bread = +1).

Average Daily Scores for Different Patterns

	Usual U.S.	Phase I	Phase II	Phase III
Negative score	-22	-9	-5	-2
Positive score	+4	+10	+13	+16
Net score	-18	+1	+8	+14

You are now ready to devise an action plan for Phase II. This action plan should follow the A, B, C sequence recommended for
Phase I: Allow three months for Block A, reducing your intake of
fatty and sugary foods; two months for Block B, reducing salt intake;
and two months for Block C, further reducing intake of HCD foods.

In Block A of Phase II undertake some of the following projects,
using two-week self-contracting periods as in Phase I: (1) Increase
intake of whole-grained breads and decrease meat intake. (2) Develop and practice meatless menu dishes (refer to natural foods
cookbooks and learn more about meatless dishes in other cuisines).
(3) Establish a routine of one or two meatless days per week. (4) Devise alternative food substitutions for specific meals, snacks, and
desserts. For each of these projects, build self-reward and social support into your plan.

In Block B create self-contracts to carry you through the needed
changes. Avoid salty foods when eating out and be selective when
using convenience foods. Label reading is of some help, but the ab-
solute amounts of salt per portion cannot be discerned from labels.
Since canned soups and vegetables are, in general, heavily salted,
seek out low-salt or no-salt-added canned goods. (As your taste buds
may not yet be prepared for this absence of salt, you may wish to
add other seasonings and minute amounts of salt to these products.)

In Block C, work to bring about the specific changes for HCD food
and alcohol control, using the same methods as in Phase I. Reduce
your intake of HCD foods to seven a day. If alcohol control is a problem, return to Chapter 4 to practice stress management skills. Use a
Deep Muscle and Mental Relaxation Drill twice daily to redirect your
urge for alcohol (especially if you drink to reduce tension). As in
Phase I, evaluate your progress at regular intervals. See how the eating pattern you have achieved after seven months of Phase II com-

pares with your targeted goals. In the next five months, consolidate your gains and work on special problems. Maintain and further your progress by insuring that the flavors of your new foods are satisfying. Use self-reward and work to maintain ongoing social support. At the end of the one-year Phase II period, record your eating pattern for a few days, using the Simplified Food-Scoring System described on pages 135-136. Your daily scores should now net approximately +8 (consisting of about 5 negative points and 13 positive points). Keep a food diary to record this data. Make a contingency contract in which you will reward yourself after you have achieved a weekly net score of +40 or more for two successive weeks. If you are so inclined, devise simple graphs to show your progress.

By the end of Phase II, you should be in excellent shape. Your risk-factor scores will have fallen to the one-point level in the weight, blood pressure, and blood cholesterol categories. You will have greatly reduced your chances of developing heart disease and even certain types of cancer. What's more, you will be enjoying healthy foods and tasting their natural flavors unadulterated by excessive amounts of sugar and salt. You will no longer be obtaining most of your protein from fat-laden animal sources. Your food bills will be dramatically reduced, and your whole family will benefit from a saner eating style.

PHASE III

Some of you will now wish to proceed to Phase III, in which about two-thirds of your protein intake is derived from vegetable sources and one-third or less from animal sources (the reverse of the usual American diet). This is a semi-vegetarian food pattern and contains all needed nutritional elements (some animal foods are needed to supply vitamin B_{12}). In Phase III vegetable protein is derived principally from legume sources with additional high-quality protein obtained from nuts, seeds, whole-grained cereals, and vegetables (the potato, for example, contains 8 percent protein). Sugar intake is derived principally from fruits and from small amounts of honey; total sugar intake is reduced to 10 percent or less of total calories (24 percent is the average in the usual American diet). Fat intake decreases to about 20 percent of calories (the U.S. average is about 40 percent) and the saturated-fat component decreases to only 3 percent of calories (the U.S. average is about 15 percent). Depending on weight-control goals, the reduced calorie intake is partially or fully replaced by complex carbohydrates, which supply about 55 percent of calories (the U.S. average is 22 percent). Salt intake is lowered to about two and one-half grams or less per day (the U.S. average is 12 grams). Although the most striking benefit of the Phase III food pattern is the prevention of cardiovascular disease, there are many secondary benefits: a decreased likelihood of developing cancer of the colon, rectum, or breast; a decrease in body weight; a decrease in dental caries; a decrease in constipation and hemorrhoids; a decrease in the severity of diabetes and other diseases associated with obesity.

In my view, the Phase III food pattern is optimal. Your palate's sensitivity is heightened because of a further decrease in exposure to sugar and salt pollution and a continued exploration of natural flavors of the Mediterranean basin and other areas. The Phase III changes follow:

PHASE III CHANGES

A. Saturated-Fat and Cholesterol Control
   1. Reduce servings of cheese (other than low-fat varieties), red meat, egg yolks, ice cream, and milk (other than nonfat) to a combined total of five per week.
   2. Continue to be alert to hidden sources of saturated fat in restaurant meals, commercial baked goods, and convenience foods.

B. Sugar Control
   1. Use fruits or fruit/nut combinations as your predominant dessert fare. Experiment with combinations of dried or fresh fruits, nuts, and whole-grained cereals for breakfast, lunch, and snacks.
   2. Use small amounts of honey in place of table sugar.

C. Salt and Caffeine Control
   1. Continue to seek out and eliminate hidden sources of excess salt.
   2. Eliminate use of salt in cooking, except on rare occasions.
   3. Eliminate use of convenience foods, except on rare occasions.
   4. Drink no more than two cups of coffee or tea a day. Continue to use herbal teas.

D. Complex-Carbohydrate and Fiber Control
   1. Have at least seven servings a day of fruit, vegetables, whole-grained or lightly milled cereals (brown rice, whole wheat, bulgur, and couscous), and legumes. Experiment with new recipes using such foods.

2. Drink fruit juices with pulp.

E. High-Caloric-Density Food Control
  1. Reduce intake of HCD foods to four or five a day. These foods should be drawn mainly from vegetable sources, preferably from whole foods such as avocados, seeds, and nuts (including unsalted, natural peanut butter).

F. Alcohol Control
  1. Maintain your alcohol consumption at 5 percent or less of your total caloric intake, as in Phases I and II.

Begin your Phase III plan by checking your cardiovascular risk score (see pages 38-39). You can proceed through Phase III as a seasoned veteran conducting what is basically a cleanup program. Employ the methods that you used in Phases I and II. Aim to achieve an average daily food point score of 14 to 18 positive points, usually with 2 or fewer negative points, with an average net score of 12 to 16 (use the Simplified Food-Scoring System described on pages 135-136). Build self-reward into your program to provide an extra push. Continue to find new books to provide interesting recipes for your alternative foods. Concentrate on making changes in one area at a time, as you did in Phases I and II (use the Block A, B, and C blueprint).

Maintenance of your new eating patterns is not difficult in your home setting but does present challenges when you eat out. If you detect a tendency to slip back to earlier patterns, call upon your repertoire of self-directed change skills to devise solutions. Maintaining your new food pattern is made easier by making sure your new habits are pleasurable. Remind yourself that you are steering a prudent course, and protect yourself against any negativistic sniping you may encounter. Continue your self-education in nutrition.

Weight control is intimately intertwined with the transformation in your food pattern. Changes in food habits mesh naturally and comfortably with efforts to achieve weight control. The weight-control methods presented in the next chapter facilitate calorie control and provide solutions to a wide variety of eating problems and urges.

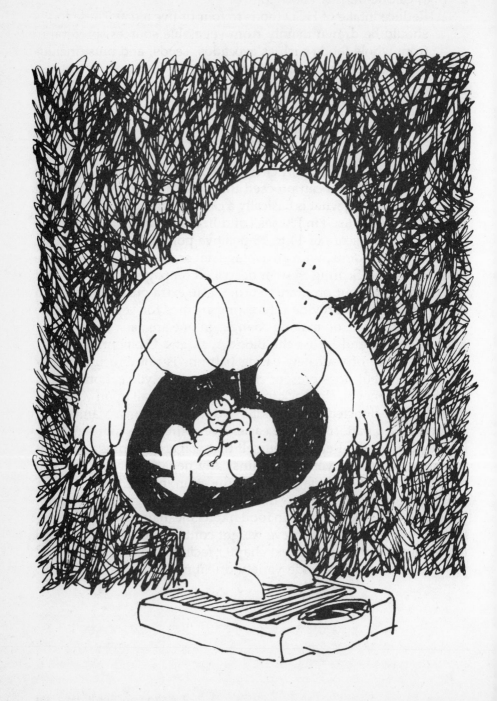

7 WEIGHT CONTROL

I f you were to think of a stereotype of the "typical American," chances are you would not include obesity in that picture. Yet Americans, gaining an average of one to two pounds a year from ages 20 to 50, are heavier than are the citizens of any other major nation. Despite the advent of a national obsession with slimness, we are not winning the weight battle. Although slimness alone obviously does not guarantee good health, the benefits of being slim are great. In my view, an effective attack on the problem of weight control would contribute as much to cardiovascular disease prevention as would any other single change in health habits.

Losing excess weight can help lower blood pressure and blood cholesterol as well as encourage you to be physically more active (which brings further benefits to cardiovascular health). Other aspects of health are also adversely affected by being overweight. Even a slight degree of overweight aggravates existing diabetes (and can trigger the onset of diabetes in a genetically susceptible person). Moderate to severe overweight can also lead to gall bladder disease, arthritis of weight-bearing joints (osteoarthritis), and to a decreased wound-healing capacity following surgery. Severe obesity can bring about decreased functioning of the lungs, leading to shortness of breath, which in turn can lead to sleep disorders.

There is often a very poor fit between cultural ideals and good health, but the American ideal of being thin is a healthy one. Plump or fat Americans usually want to be thinner and will try an almost inexhaustible variety of special diets to lose weight (usually along the lines of "the quicker the better"). Most people are familiar with temporary success while on strict diets, but the lost weight is all too often regained after they resume their previous eating patterns.

THE RHYTHM METHOD OF GIRTH CONTROL

This cycle of gaining, losing, and regaining weight is as American as apple pie. The experience of initial success and ultimate failure is a tremendous frustration and a significant cardiovascular burden for millions of people who are aided and abetted by the "quick-weight-loss" industry. Fad diets, crash programs, quick cures, promises to "roll away the inches" are generally useless for *long-term* weight control; frequently they are harmful. Low-carbohydrate or high-protein diets, for instance, are almost always high in animal fat, and can result in elevated blood cholesterol (or in attacks of gout). Starvation methods can precipitate gouty attacks as well as upset the fluid, mineral, and protein balance of the body; they should *never* be used without close medical supervision.

Virtually every year for the past 20 years, the American public has been treated to a new miracle cure for overweight. One of the most recent, the liquid protein diet, is no new medical breakthrough. It has long been known that people will lose weight while on liquid diets. But a liquid protein diet can be extremely dangerous. Even when conducted under close medical supervision, there are indications that such a diet can cause disturbances in the body's potassium balance and can lead to ketosis, an abnormal build-up of acids in the body tissues. Serious cardiac arrhythmias have also been reported, and some of these have resulted in fatalities. Weight losses from other shortcuts such as jaw wiring, diet pills, or fasting are usually temporary because, again, they do not change the underlying habits that cause the weight problem. The mere act of "going on a diet" implies that one will eventually "go off."

If you have followed this "rhythm" method of dieting, you have ample reason to be interested in an entirely different approach. Applying methods of self-directed change to weight problems provides an effective way to achieve *permanent* weight control. Using these methods, you will avoid the unpleasant, potentially harmful eating patterns known as diets. Instead you will devise a program that allows you gradually to change the habits that make you gain weight. This program should constitute a permanent, pleasurable change in your life-style. It need not be arbitrary or authoritarian in its design; you will make the important decisions about your specific weight-loss goals and the way to attain them. This chapter will provide the framework and a variety of methods to make the process work for you.

IS THIS PROGRAM MEANT FOR ME?

If you are thinking of skimming over this chapter, don't. Statistically speaking, it is extremely likely that weight loss is a subject that is—or will be—highly relevant to your own health and well-being. Between 80 and 90 percent of all adults in the U.S. are at least 5 percent over their ideal weight. Overweight is so common in our culture that relative plumpness is often accepted as the healthy standard and the lean individual may be considered unusual or too skinny. Many people regard themselves as "normal, healthy adults" despite having gained 20 to 30 pounds since the age of 20. Such a weight gain is not normal; it is merely typical. Almost all adults would be healthier if they were to lose *at least* two-thirds of the weight gained after age 20. Even people who currently carry no excess weight can profit from the methods presented here in order to prevent future weight gain (this includes young adults just beginning their typical weight gain and dieters who have already lost their desired pounds and now want to keep them off).

THE NEW GIRTH-CONTROL METHOD

Let me begin by reassuring readers who are battle-scarred from unsuccessful diets and are wary of experiencing more frustration that what you will find in this chapter is *not* another diet; instead, you will be formulating permanent changes in your life-style at a rate you find pleasant. The complexity of methods needed to achieve weight control will vary, depending on personal factors. Some people will need to change only a few habits to solve problems of weight gain. To bring about desired changes, you will progress through the following six stages: (1) identifying your degree of overweight and your barriers to action; (2) building your commitment, enlisting social support from family, friends, associates, and/or organized weight-loss or exercise groups; (3) developing an awareness of the factors that influence your eating and exercise habits; (4) devising and implementing an action plan using behavioral rehearsal, imagery, self-reward, environmental planning, and other skills of self-directed change; (5) evaluating and adjusting your plan as needed; and (6) maintaining your progress and guarding against setbacks.

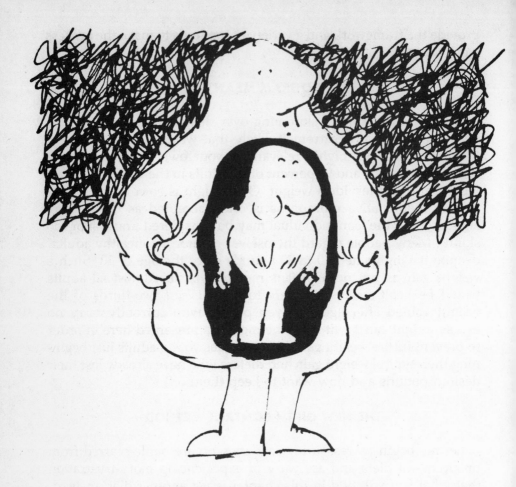

ONE: IDENTIFYING THE PROBLEM

Identifying weight-control problems has three facets: (1) determining the amount of excess weight; (2) determining the impact of this excess on your total cardiovascular risk level; and (3) determining your underlying attitudes toward weight reduction. To gauge whether and/or to what extent you are overweight, use the simple formula introduced in Chapter 3: for women, ideal weight = (height in inches × 3.5) − 108; for men, ideal weight = (height in inches × 4) − 128.

This formula for calculating ideal weight may not work for some people; small-boned individuals with slight builds or large-boned individuals with muscular builds will need supplementary methods. Unless you were overweight as a young adult, your weight at age 20 will provide a good approximation of your ideal weight. If you were already overweight by age 20 and have subsequently gained additional weight, a return to your earlier weight would still be a considerable achievement. Another valuable method to determine your degree of overweight is a skinfold pinch test. Press together about an inch of flesh at your side, at waist level just above the hip bone. If the skinfold is wider than the width of your thumb, then you are probably at least ten pounds over your ideal weight. If it is about the width of your index finger, you are about five to ten pounds overweight. If it is the width of your little finger, you belong to the 3 to 5 percent minority of truly slender Americans.

To determine your weight-related cardiovascular risk level, use the following system: ideal weight=0 points; 1-9 pounds excess=1 point; 10-19 pounds excess=2 points; 20-29 pounds excess=3 points; 30 or more pounds excess=4 points. Next determine your total cardiovascular risk score as gauged from the Simplified Self-Scoring Test of Chronic Disease Risk on pages 38-39 of Chapter 3.

By reducing your weight, you can also lower your risk in all the other risk areas except smoking. Weight loss will lower blood pressure (especially if you also decrease your salt intake) and blood cholesterol (especially if you cut down on foods high in animal fat). The increased physical activity most people need to achieve weight control will readily decrease risk associated with a sedentary lifestyle. Many people will find that the stress management skills developed as a part of a weight-control plan will also lower stress-related cardiovascular risk.

Even if you know you should lose weight, you may feel that you simply can't do it, or that you can't keep the pounds from coming back. At this point, it is extremely important to examine your thinking to see whether any of the following beliefs (or myths) about losing weight act as barriers to your commitment:

1. "I have a glandular condition." Some people think that glandular problems involving thyroid deficiency are responsible for overweight. This is a myth. Overweight is *not* caused by thyroid deficiency. Careful research, such as the excellent studies carried out by Dr. Edward Rynearson of the Mayo Clinic, has shown that people with low thyroid function are no more overweight than their brothers and sisters whose thyroid levels are normal.

2. "It's normal to gain weight as you get older." Wrong! In less developed countries, where sedentary life-styles and Western food habits have yet to arrive, adults generally *lose* weight as they grow older (due to the normal loss of muscle mass that occurs with age).

People should not gain weight after age 20, especially since even a constant weight from ages 30 to 60 in fact indicates an *increase* in fat tissue because of muscle loss during that time.

3. "Fatness runs in my family." When overweight runs in families, it is related to the fact that family eating habits are passed from one generation to the next as well as to a true genetic influence. For example, identical twins reared apart conform to the weight of their natural parents more closely than to that of their adoptive parents. Although such evidence in support of a genetic basis for overweight is present, the environmental effect is also strong. The most convincing role of environment is seen in migrating populations. For example, as Japanese migrate to Hawaii and then to California, average body weights steadily increase, especially in those Japanese who quickly adopt the eating patterns of their host country.

4. "Exercise increases my appetite." Moderate or vigorous exercise usually reduces the appetite for a short period of time, and mild exercise distracts you from idle snacking. Exercise can be used effectively to suppress eating urges. Athletes or people who engage in heavy physical labor do have larger appetites, but such individuals may expend 500 or 1,000 calories per day in exercise and hence can eat more than less active peers while still remaining in caloric balance.

5. "It's no use; I always regain my weight." Unfortunately, this is a common experience for people who are overweight. It is important to realize how strongly you are influenced by social learning (your childhood eating habits) and your environment. No one is *ordained* to be overweight. Applying concrete methods of self-directed change to your weight-control problem supplies you with better and more diverse tools to achieve permanent change than you have had before, when relying on willpower or temporary diets.

6. "It's my metabolism; I gain weight on practically no calories." This is a common belief that needs to be examined rationally. Some moderately overweight people may consume fewer calories than other individuals of normal weight. In such cases, physical activity is usually the determining variable; overweight people generally are less physically active than are their thinner counterparts. For everyone, body weight is the consequence of a *balance* between *energy consumed* (caloric intake) and *energy expended*. Even if you gain weight on fewer calories than do your friends, the "in balances out" rule still applies. Your metabolic rate may slow down slightly as you grow older, but this merely means that you need either to consume

fewer calories or to expend more. Weight gain is *not* a necessary consequence.

7. "Pills or shots to cut down on hunger really work." Pills, like special diets and jaw wiring, are but temporary window dressing since they do nothing to alter the habits that cause overweight. Although they may accelerate the early phase of weight loss, diet pills have potentially harmful side effects and can become addictive.

8. "Losing weight isn't worth giving up all my favorite foods and disrupting my family life." Losing weight doesn't have to be disruptive or unpleasant. The basic point to realize is that you must lose weight in a comfortable, pleasant manner or else you'll revert back to previous habits.

Do any of the above belief barriers embody attitudes of your own? Dredge up the underlying beliefs that may inhibit your success. Bringing such attitudes into the open allows you to examine them objectively. Monitor your thoughts about losing weight for a week or two and make a list of your negative beliefs. Counter your list of negative thoughts with objective, rational alternatives that you record and then practice at least twice daily for a week or so.

TWO: BUILDING COMMITMENT

Changing deep-rooted habits that result in overweight requires effort and organization. To augment your commitment to change, it is helpful to take a rather formal first step, such as writing a self-contract—a statement of your intent to plan a program of weight control. Tell others of your intent and involve them in your plans.

You may wish to work with a friend or spouse as a helper or participant. An ideal situation is for the helper to work on behavior-change efforts of his or her own as well. A further step might include joining a health club, gym, or group such as Weight Watchers, Take Off Pounds Sensibly (TOPS), or Overeaters Anonymous to supplement your own efforts. Alternatively, you might want to create your own group to work on the self-directed change principles presented in this book.

THREE: INCREASING AWARENESS
OF BEHAVIOR PATTERNS

If you are overweight, you need to change either your eating or your exercise patterns—or, as is almost always the case, both. To determine the roots of your weight problem, keep a food and exer-

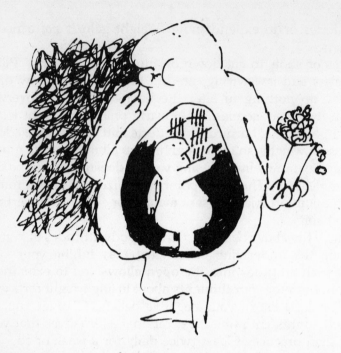

cise diary for two weeks before you formulate a specific plan for losing weight. An example of such a diary appears on page 149.

Diagnosis of Sample Diary. The person in our sample diary had seven snacks and three meals during the course of the day. Nearly all snacks were of high caloric density (glazed doughnut, cheese, sugar and cream added to coffee, cookies). Only three times did the person primarily socialize while eating. During five of the eating episodes, the person focused on some other activity—work, television, dinner preparation. Meals were often eaten hurriedly. The individual's exercise level was extremely low. Self-diagnosis thus reveals: (1) too many snacks, (2) too many high-caloric-density foods, (3) too little exercise,(4) engaging in other activities while eating, and (5) eating too fast.

You may prefer separate diaries for food and exercise, or you may wish to add other information (e.g., using the knowledge gained from Chapter 6, you could classify foods according to their caloric density). Approximate the time spent eating meals, snacking, etc. Also wear a pedometer during this period in order to gauge accurately the number of miles you walk per day. After collecting this information you will know far more precisely what your problem habits are: where and how many times you snack or eat a meal, how fast you eat, what else you do while eating, and whether or not you

FOOD AND EXERCISE DIARY

Day of Week and Date: _____   Name: _____

Time of day	What did I eat or do?	Where?	Time spent eating or exercising?	What else did I do while eating?
7:30 A.M.	Ate breakfast: coffee, sugar, 3 slices of bacon, 2 eggs, whole milk	Kitchen table	10 min.	Talked
8:30 A.M.	Coffee, sugar, cream	Office		Worked
10:30 A.M.	Coffee, sugar, cream, glazed doughnut	Office		Worked
12:00 NOON	Lunch: chopped sirloin, buttered vegetables, roll and butter, chocolate cake	Restaurant: lunch meeting	15 min.	Talked
2:30 P.M.	Walked	To meeting	5 min.	
2:45 P.M.	Coffee, sugar, cream	Meeting	10 min.	
3:30 P.M.	Soft drink	Delicatessen	10 min.	Talked
6:00 P.M.	Tasted and nibbled various things	Kitchen area	15 min.	Prepared dinner
6:30 P.M.	Drank two cocktails and ate cheese and crackers	TV room	30 min.	Watched TV news
7:00 P.M.	Dinner: steak, frozen peas, baked potato with butter and sour cream, ice cream	TV room	20 min.	Watched TV and talked
10:00 P.M.	Checked pedometer: walked 1½ miles			
11:00 P.M.	Had 6 cookies and a glass of whole milk	Bedroom	5 min.	Watched TV

eat a large number of high-caloric-density foods. (Precise description of foods is unnecessary.) Such a diary provides the raw data for an accurate self-diagnosis. Having identified the basic problems, you are then ready to devise ways to alter these habits. Inspect your eating and exercise diary to identify your own foibles.

Food Thoughts

In addition to keeping a food and exercise diary to provide you with information about the external cues associated with eating, it is helpful to keep a food thoughts diary to alert you to the internal cues that trigger eating. For example, binge eating can result from setting perfectionistic goals ("I won't ever eat cake again after today") and unduly self-critical thoughts following any deviation from them ("I don't have any willpower; I may as well have another piece"). Overeating may also occur in response to emotional factors—stress, tension, loneliness, boredom, depression, etc. For a period of a week or two, record the thoughts that precede snacking or eating of problem foods. Then counter them with specific, rational alternatives. Your list of thoughts that trigger eating (derived from your food thoughts diary) and of substitute countering thoughts might look something like this:

Thoughts That Trigger Eating	Substitute Countering Thoughts
1. I'm nervous; I need a drink and a snack to relax.	1. My new skills in relaxation are more effective than liquor or food in helping me to unwind.
2. I don't have the willpower to stay away from second helpings.	2. Putting the unused food away before I sit down to eat is a simple preventive measure.
3. I'm not losing weight. I'm a failure.	3. I must expect minor setbacks. This isn't a catastrophe. I'm gradually learning ways to change habits that are causing my problem.
4. (fill in) _____ _____	4. (fill in) _____ _____
5. (fill in) _____ _____	5. (fill in) _____ _____

At least twice a day for about a week, practice substituting these confidence-building countering thoughts in place of negative thoughts expressing frustration, anger, etc. Role-play your most self-critical ruminations and then vigorously dispute yourself in turn.

FOUR: BUILDING AN ACTION PLAN

You have now gained experience in detecting problems that are apt to be troublesome in your weight-control efforts. When you embark on your action plan, be sure to incorporate techniques that reinforce your sense of accomplishment and your resolve to continue. An action plan for weight control should ideally be developed in conjunction with an action plan for adopting the alternative food pattern described in Chapter 6. These two programs are intimately intertwined; do not view your weight-control efforts in isolation from larger changes in your eating patterns. An ideal sequence for combining the two programs is to develop your action plan for weight control to coincide with the beginning of Block C (high-caloric-density food and alcohol control) of Phase I of the alternative food pattern.

The best motto for weight loss is "the slower the better." This is bound to be initially unpopular, because most overweight people yearn for instant transformation. But the key to success in permanent weight loss is contained in a simple principle: *Unless you build new habits and become comfortable with them as you shed your pounds, you will regain the pounds eventually. You have to be able to live with the new program and enjoy it.* You may feel heroic, martyred, and proud as you starve yourself on grapefruit, cottage cheese, and all the celery you can eat, but unless you've changed your habits so gradually that you *enjoy* the alterations that you are bringing about, you won't win over the long haul. Even if you lose weight rapidly, you will feel that you are being deprived and you will find your self-denying program unpleasant.

Set a goal of losing *no more than four pounds a month* during the first six months of your weight-control program. (An initial loss of two to three pounds of water may occur during the first week, so up to a six-pound weight loss may be a reasonable goal during the first month.) Individuals who have only about ten pounds to lose may decide to lose less rapidly. Many people find that a slow weight loss occurs automatically after embarking on an exercise program.

The key to goal setting is flexibility. You will determine your own rate of progress and will be able, with experience, to know how much weight you can lose without feeling strained or uncomfortable. Don't rush yourself. If it took decades to develop the habits that cause weight problems, then even two or three years is not too long a time to achieve a significant and permanent change in your weight.

The problem-solving sections in the remainder of this chapter will give you more specifics about how to change your eating style, how to achieve recommended reductions in your intake of high-caloric-density foods, and how to suppress eating urges.

Solving Eating-Style Problems

I will now discuss seven common eating-style problems and their solutions. Each could be tackled through a separate two-week self-contract plan.

1. *Eating rapidly.* Eating rapidly does not allow sufficient time for the stomach to sense the presence of food and for the digestive process to allow your blood sugar to increase and signal the appetite center in the brain when you are no longer hungry. Accordingly, by eating rapidly you run the risk of overeating. To become more aware of your eating speed, ask a friend or family member to alert you to abnormally rapid eating. Consciously slow down while eating; don't allow time pressures to overpower you at meals. Relax and enjoy your food.

2. *High-calorie snacks.* Phase out your intake of high-calorie snack foods. Do not make them readily available between meals. Eat low-calorie substitutes (such as fresh vegetables) for snacks.

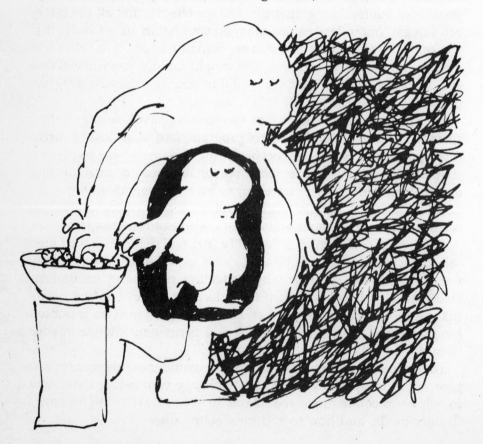

3. *Surplus food at meals.* Decide how much food will be served at the beginning of a meal. Each individual in the family can still have a say in how much he or she wants, but the remaining food should not be left on the table where it becomes a temptation. Parents should not eat the food left on children's plates.

4. *Buying food on an empty stomach.* Do not go grocery shopping when you are hungry. This will help you avoid buying high-calorie problem foods. The first two hours after any meal is the best time for grocery shopping. Let your shopping list and not your appetite be your guide.

5. *Avoiding problem foods.* Keeping problem foods out of the house can help you avoid needless temptation. It is important to have the family agree on this matter. Phase down gradually so that no one feels deprived. Substitute foods that are enjoyable, more healthful, and less fattening.

6. *Where you eat.* Each place where you commonly eat becomes associated in your subconscious mind with food. Merely entering these areas can thus trigger subliminal thoughts about food—and a desire to eat—even when you are not hungry. Limit most of your home eating to one or two places (e.g., the dining room and kitchen tables). This helps to limit the number of areas in your home that your subconscious links with food.

7. *Avoiding non-food-related activities while eating.* When your attention is diverted by other activities—watching television, working, reading, etc.—you run the risk of "unconscious eating." By focusing on the tastes and aromas of the foods you are eating, you become more conscious of your appetite and whether or not you are truly hungry. Do you eat popcorn at a movie just because you love popcorn? Do you sometimes munch on food while watching TV when you aren't really hungry? What activities trigger your desire to eat? Once you locate them, consciously avoid eating while engaging in those activities.

Solving Calorie-Control Problems

For many people calorie control is the most important eating problem. By reducing the number of snacks and the number of high-caloric-density foods you eat, you can greatly reduce your calorie intake. It is also important, however, to use methods of self-directed change to suppress urges for high-caloric-density foods. Calorie control and control of blood cholesterol and blood pressure go hand in hand (many high-caloric-density foods are also high in saturated fat and cholesterol and/or salt). This means that some of the nutritional knowledge needed to identify high-caloric-density foods is achieved by mastering the saturated-fat and salt discussions in Chapter 6. Hence, if you have begun Phase I of the alternative food pattern, you have already begun to restrict some of your high-caloric-density foods.

The most common way of teaching calorie control asks people to learn the caloric content of numerous foods, usually by referring to lengthy tables listing calories per portion size. In the table on pages 114-115, Chapter 6, I gave you instead a single list of common foods classified into categories of high, medium, and low caloric density. I suggest that you use this simple chart as your basic tool for achieving calorie control. (For most people, this simple method of calorie counting will suffice. If you prefer to augment this with more complex methods of calorie counting, feel free to refer to calorie tables.)

Armed with your awareness of the caloric density of the foods you eat, inspect your food and exercise diary to determine the number of HCD foods that you consume per day. The basic scoring unit is a "usual portion." (The average American eats about 15 HCD foods a day.) Your record for the week might look like this:

HIGH-CALORIC-DENSITY FOODS: WEEK ONE

	M	T	W	Th	F	Sa	Su	Daily Average
Number HCD foods per day	15	14	15	15	14	18	17	15

Let's assume that your average is close to 15 per day and that you intend to focus on reducing your intake of HCD foods as your next weight-control effort. The self-contract that follows shows how you might proceed.

SELF-CONTRACT FOR REDUCING INTAKE OF HIGH-CALORIC-DENSITY FOODS

During the next two weeks I plan to reduce my consumption of HCD foods from my current average of 15 a day to 10 a day. I will focus especially on my intake of HCD snack foods. My helper will be _____. My responsibilities will be (1) to record my daily intake of HCD foods (I will use my diary to keep track of this) and (2) to reward myself and my helper each weekend that I reach my goal. My helper's responsibilities will be (1) to help me cut down on eating HCD foods and (2) to encourage me, during meals we eat together, to follow my plan.

Date: _____ Signed: _____

Review date: _____ Helper: _____

A week after making this initial plan, review it to see whether you need to make revisions. It may take several months to attain satisfactory control of your intake of HCD foods if your food patterns require considerable modification. Changes will occur most satisfactorily if the entire family is actively involved. If this is to be a family effort, then devise family rewards for successfully reaching targeted goals.

Solving Problems of Emotionally Induced Eating

Many people have weight-control problems that are linked to their internal thinking environments. Such people may be quite reasonable in their eating habits except during periods when they are anxious, depressed, bored, under severe stress, etc.

There are four general ways of dealing with this problem: (1) environmental control (e.g., limiting the availability of and exposure to problem foods); (2) general stress management (e.g., practicing deep muscle relaxation and mental relaxation—see Chapter 4); (3) retraining mental processes to overcome problems of emotionally induced eating (e.g., devising confidence-building drills to substitute rational counterthoughts in place of the negative thoughts that often precede problem eating); and (4) special procedures to suppress eating urges (e.g., practicing an urge-suppression drill when thinking cues evoke eating urges).

Restricting the availability of problem foods may not always eliminate your cravings for them. Because of the strength of the emotionally induced stimulus to eat, you will need specific methods to decrease urges that break through your defenses.

In Chapter 4, you learned about behavioral rehearsal drills as a means of coping with stress and tension. To increase your skill in suppressing eating urges, I suggest you practice the following drill every day for at least a week or two, and then periodically as needed:

BEHAVIORAL REHEARSAL DRILL FOR
SUPPRESSING EATING URGES

1. In a quiet room, sit or lie down in a comfortable position. Think of a food that you particularly crave in response to emotional cues. Bring this image into your mind so that you actually feel an urge to eat the food. (It may take a while to master this technique.)

2. Next, imagine an unpleasant sensation connected with food (e.g., a very bitter taste in your mouth). If this reduces your urge to eat the food, then go to the next step. If the urge persists unabated, think of one of the following: feeling nauseous, being overweight, or having dirt and sand mixed in with your food. Practice your imagery training so that you become proficient.

3. Assuming that you have partly or completely suppressed the eating urge by coupling it with a negative image, complete the urge-suppression drill by using a Muscle Relaxation/Mental Relaxation Drill or an Instant Relaxation Drill (see Chapter 4).

4. After successfully suppressing your eating urge, reward yourself. Deep muscle relaxation, though used as an urge suppressant, is also the beginning of a self-reward sequence (as is the peaceful imagery in the mental relaxation phase). You may find it effective to envision yourself successfully refusing an offer of the problem food or looking slender and attractive. Rehearse mentally a positive self-statement. Another reward could be to engage in a pleasurable activity. Or you might record 1 point for every successful urge suppression and reward yourself for specific point totals (e.g., entertainment, 10 points; dinner out, 15 points, etc.). Use your ingenuity in devising diverse rewards—symbolic and material, immediate and delayed.

After mastering this drill you will be equipped to use an abbreviated version for suppressing eating urges that arise spontaneously. Such urges can trap the unwary. Therefore, practice shortened versions of the drill during the day—at home, at work, etc. Rapidly conjure the eating urge, then think of a negative image, and follow this with an Instant Relaxation Drill. After you have practiced these quick sequences you can adapt them to counter unexpected urges for problem foods. An alternative method to suppress eating urges is to take a brief walk or engage in some other form of exercise.

Solving Exercise Problems

Sedentary living habits are a major cause of overweight. If you are relatively sedentary (your pedometer readings and aerobic exercise levels are low), then refer to Chapter 5 and coordinate an exercise action plan with other components of your weight-control program.

FIVE: EVALUATING YOUR ACTION PLAN

Pause at regular intervals during your action plan to evaluate whether or not you need to return to earlier phases of your program (identifying problems, building commitment, or increasing awareness). Evaluate your progress and determine what special problems need attention. The graph below is an example of how you might record the results of a plan to reduce snacking.

SIX: MAINTAINING YOUR WEIGHT-CONTROL PROGRAM

As you proceed on your weight-loss program, you will need to expend effort to maintain and further your progress. Although your new habits can offer you a more pleasant life-style than you previously experienced, you must protect against relapses. Hazards to successful maintenance include (1) weakness in social support, (2) weakness in self-reward, (3) unanticipated personal life changes, (4) problems related to eating out, entertaining, being entertained,

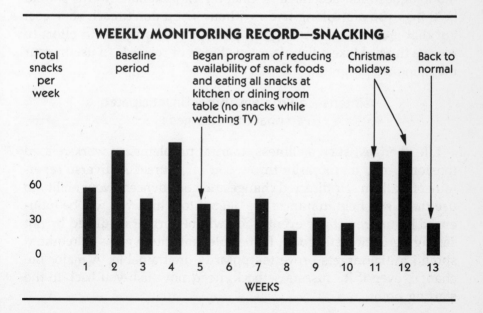

WEEKLY MONITORING RECORD—SNACKING

and (5) unanticipated eating urges. I will address these issues separately.

Maintenance Problem One: Weakness in Social Support

During your action plan, you may have involved family members and friends in your efforts. As the novelty wears off, their involvement may fade. The solution to this problem lies in your recognition that social support is still necessary and in your continued efforts to engage others in your program. Devise ways to achieve such involvement.

Maintenance Problem Two: Weakness in Self-Reward

Of all the methods used in self-directed change, I find people are most reluctant to use self-reward. I believe this reluctance stems from our cultural background—the Puritan ethic and our Judeo-Christian heritage. Reward yourself for your progress. Such rewards can take four forms: (1) pleasurable activities, (2) positive statements about yourself, (3) symbolic rewards, and (4) material rewards. Pleasurable activities include physical exercise, deep muscle relaxation, mental relaxation, and the use of positive imagery. Positive self-statements are generated to counter negative thoughts in your self-monologues (first described in Chapter 4). Material rewards should be things you are willing to do without if you don't reach your goal but that are attractive enough to prompt you to put forth effort to receive them. Make a list of various kinds of rewards to use in your maintenance program.

Maintenance Problem Three: Unanticipated Personal Life Changes

Life changes, such as illness, marital problems, or work-related tensions, may temporarily throw you off course. A diverse repertoire of skills in self-directed change and confidence in your ability to use them will help minimize the degree to which you will be influenced by unpredictable events. You will be further insulated by not setting perfectionistic goals. Be flexible; substitute goals as required should initial targets prove temporarily unattainable. A major life change, even if it causes a setback, need not push you back to the starting point.

Maintenance Problem Four: Eating Out, Entertaining, Being Entertained

Be moderate. When entertaining, or being entertained, exercise simple restraint and limit your intake of high-caloric-density foods. Don't allow a misplaced sense of social decorum to put supposed feelings of friends above your own welfare. You needn't turn up your nose at high-cholesterol, high-caloric-density foods that your host or hostess may serve, but neither need you "inhale" them with abandon. True friends will respect your wishes—and your refusals of seconds.

Maintenance Problem Five: Unanticipated Eating Cues

You walk by a candy shop or a bakery. You see your favorite "fat treat" on the menu of a fine restaurant. What to do? Cue-alienation and urge-suppression methods will be of much benefit. Still, you can allow yourself an occasional high-calorie treat; just don't overdo.

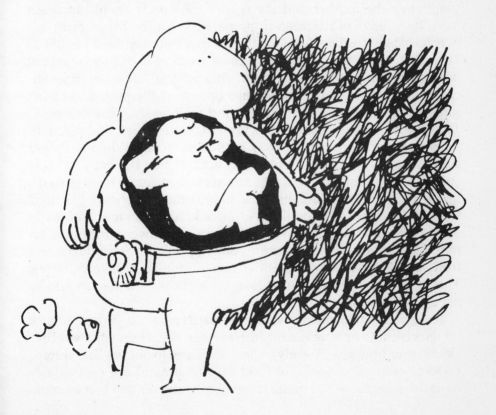

Maintenance Problem Six: Inadequate Commitment

Recent research has shown that "contingency contracting" can furnish a strong additional boost to change efforts. This system involves making a self-contract which specifies that you will deposit a particular sum of money or a valued possession with a spouse or helper. The self-contract also specifies that the money or goods will be returned only if you succeed in attaining certain goals. If, for example, you succeed in losing ten pounds in six months, you might arrange for return of $10 a month for each of the next six months if you maintain this or a lower weight. If you do not maintain your goal, the money or belongings must be donated to a charity of your choice. This system has the added virtue of maintaining a close connection with the helper you have chosen to manage your contingency contract.

OBESITY PREVENTION IN CHILDREN

Obesity prevention should truly begin at the beginning; during pregnancy the mother and the rest of the family should increase their knowledge of nutrition in preparation for the baby's birth.

If possible, it is beneficial for the mother to breast-feed her child. The reasons for this are many. Breast-feeding is of psychological benefit to both mother and child. In addition, breast-feeding increases resistance to childhood infections and allergies, and breast milk is markedly lower in total fat and sodium than is cow's milk. Thus the infant begins life with a normal, natural diet. Breast-fed infants in general are not as fat as bottle-fed babies. When an infant stops suckling, the mother generally accepts that her baby has had sufficient nourishment, whereas mothers often coax a baby to finish his or her bottle, thus initiating the infant's first experience of forced feeding. The second experience of forced feeding comes with early introduction of solid foods. Use of cereals between four and six months is not likely to be harmful, but egg yolk, meat products, and fruits with large amounts of added sugar are high in caloric density. They should be withheld for at least six months, and then should be used only sparingly.

Family eating habits and sedentary patterns, such as dependence on television as entertainment (the average American child watches almost four hours of TV daily), also contribute to obesity in children. Food as reward or denial of food as punishment are particularly harmful. Exercise as the mainstay of obesity prevention is even more critical for children and adolescents than for adults. Although enforced caloric restriction is never wise for young people, parents should insure that healthy low-calorie snacks are available for their children. The preventive prescription is to create a household eating and exercise life-style that is healthy for all.

Fortunately, even 40 years or more of "learning to be fat" can be reversed. For the great majority of readers, the information in this book will be sufficient. However, individuals who are more than 80 pounds overweight should seek professional guidance as well—especially if evidence of high blood pressure, high blood cholesterol or triglyceride levels, gout, or diabetes is discovered. Even the individual who is currently *not* overweight can benefit greatly from a preventive approach to weight control.

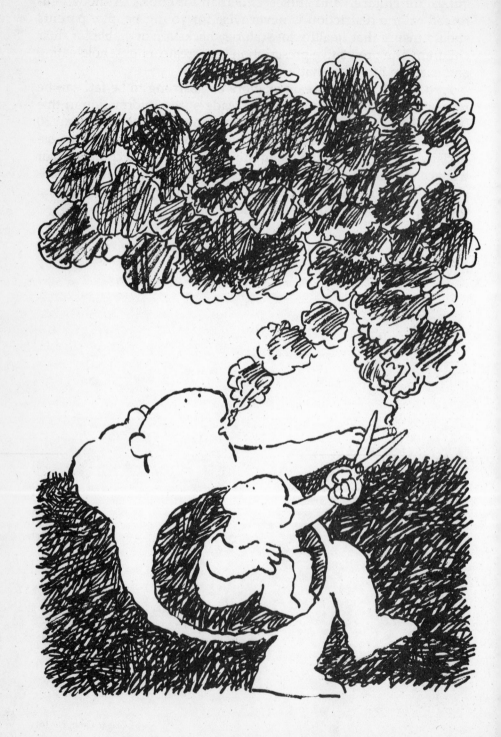

8

HOW TO STOP SMOKING

Of all the risk factors in heart disease, smoking is one of the most difficult to change. According to surveys, over two-thirds of the current 51 million smokers in the U.S. would like to quit. (Most of these smokers have tried to stop before but have failed to quit permanently.) Surveys have also shown that although essentially all adults are fully aware of the risks of lung cancer and chronic lung diseases such as emphysema incurred by smoking, fewer than half realize that smoking is a major risk factor for heart attacks and strokes—and for the promotion of the fatty arterial deposits of atherosclerosis.

Actually, the risks attributable to smoking are about three times greater for developing a heart attack than for developing lung cancer. This cardiovascular risk falls dramatically after a smoker quits; most studies indicate that the extra risk of heart attack due to smoking is cut in half within a year after quitting. However, it takes a full five to ten years before an ex-smoker reaches the lower cardiovascular and lung cancer risk level of a person who has never smoked. The lung damage of advanced emphysema is irreversible.

If you are a smoker and would like to break your habit, you should be encouraged by the fact that much of the cardiovascular damage caused by smoking is reversible, as well as by the fact that every year for the past 15 years more than one million Americans have stopped smoking.

Unfortunately, for every person who has successfully stopped smoking there are many who fail in their first serious attempt to quit and still more who fail frequently by falling into a pattern of sporadic periods of stopping and starting. If you are a smoker, prior experiences of failure may have reduced your confidence in new methods to quit. It is not helpful to share the common misconception that kicking the habit is simply a matter of "willpower." Such an attitude leads to frequent self-critical thoughts (which are harmful to efforts to quit) about one's lack of this illusive trait during particularly difficult or stressful periods.

If willpower is not the answer, what can you rely on? Learned skills—skills that allow you far greater self-control and power to shape your environment and your reactions to daily experiences. These tools will enable you to stop smoking with a far greater chance of permanent success than you would have unaided. (Experience in treatment programs has confirmed that methods of self-directed change do have a higher rate of success than an individual's unaided effort to quit his habit "cold turkey.")

If you are a smoker who has tried to quit, only to resume smoking later, these methods provide you with a broad arsenal of skills that enhance your ability to quit smoking permanently. The following techniques form a six-stage program for self-directed change: (1) identifying the problem; (2) building your confidence and commitment to quit; (3) developing an awareness of why, where, and when you smoke; (4) developing and implementing an action plan to quit smoking; (5) evaluating your plan; and (6) maintaining your ex-smoking status. For those who try and fail with the six-stage program, a second attempt can include the help of a new agent, nicotine-containing chewing gum, and its use will also be described. All of these methods have been used as a part of the program of the Stanford Center for Research in Disease Prevention.

ONE: IDENTIFYING THE PROBLEM

Begin your effort to quit smoking by finding out the degree of cardiovascular risk to assign to your smoking habit. Refer to the Simplified Self-Scoring Test of Chronic Disease Risk on pages 38-39. Smoking-related cardiovascular risk correlates directly with the number of cigarettes smoked per day (see Figure 1-4 in Chapter 1). Because cardiovascular damage is cumulative, total exposure time is also relevant. Therefore, to refine your scoring of cardiovascular risk, double your score if you have smoked a total of 15 years or more.

Although a confirmed smoker has a good idea of how much he smokes, a 20 percent underestimate is common. Also, smoking rates often vary with work habits, seasons, or the amount of stress a person is experiencing. To determine the number of cigarettes you smoke each day, keep a simple smoking diary over a period of one or two weeks.

You are then ready to examine your attitudes about quitting (and their sources) and your feelings about your capacity to quit. Identifying potential resistances to change is the most important step in becoming an ex-smoker. You can work through these blocks by actively challenging these belief barriers and replacing them with alternative attitudes. Once you have uncovered your mental blocks and have worked to counter them, actual changes in attitude occur much more readily and sometimes even automatically. The chart on the next page provides examples of common belief barriers and helpful countering views. After thinking through these examples, make a list expressing your own feelings about quitting.

After developing your own list, work on countering your belief barriers with alternative attitudes. Over a period of one or two weeks, record your negative thoughts about quitting in a small, convenient diary or notebook that you carry with you. A few times a day, when you light up or finish a cigarette, ask yourself how you feel about quitting. Practice substituting and recording alternative positive thoughts for your belief barriers. To develop these optimistic thoughts, imagine yourself as an ex-smoker. What would you say to yourself if you *were* an ex-smoker?

This is a way to bring into the open your deeply embedded resistances. Ordinarily, becoming aware of irrational negative attitudes will allow you to replace them without difficulty with rational substitute thoughts. Even if you initially believe you cannot quit, practice in countering your negative inner monologues with alternative statements will allow you to become more open-minded about your capacity to change; it will also train you to see yourself as a potential nonsmoker. It is helpful to make a self-contract to cover a two-week phase for overcoming belief barriers (see Chapters 3 and 4 for examples of written self-contracts). To make and honor such a contract may initially strike you as a burdensome task, but its results will amply reward your efforts.

Also become proficient in stress management skills (described in Chapter 4) before formally attempting to quit smoking. Skill in effective stress management will greatly increase your chances of becoming a successful ex-smoker. Physical exercise is another antidote for smoking urges. If you are quite sedentary (e.g., if your pedometer reading is less than two miles per day), you will find it

ATTITUDES THAT IMPEDE OR PROMOTE SUCCESS IN A PROGRAM TO QUIT SMOKING PERMANENTLY

Negative Belief Barriers	Effective Positive Counterarguments
1. I'm afraid I'll gain weight if I stop smoking.	1. If I begin an exercise program as part of my plan to stop smoking, I can avoid gaining weight.
2. I don't have the willpower to quit.	2. Quitting is not a mattter of willpower. Learning to kick my smoking habit is a matter of acquiring the skills that will give me greater control over my own behavior.
3. I've been smoking too long to stop.	3. It's never too late to stop; cardiovascular risk due to smoking drops dramatically after quitting.
4. I've tried and failed before, and it's too nerve-wracking to go through it again.	4. Methods of self-directed change described in this book can give me a better chance of success; they sound promising.
5. Cigarettes relieve my tension.	5. Learning stress management skills and engaging in more exercise are effective in relieving tension.
6. I enjoy smoking after a meal.	6. I have learned to associate smoking with the satisfied feeling I have after finishing a meal; I can train myself to break this artificial link between smoking and pleasant expreiences.
7. I'd rather keep smoking and take my chances. Besides, I'm healthy; I don't intend to get lung cancer or have a heart attack. I'm not an alarmist.	7. Actually, I am not so flippant about increasing my chances of dying prematurely from lung cancer or from a heart attack or stroke. I have been telling myself that it can't happen to me. It can. It's worth it to me to quit smoking.
8. (fill in) _____ _____ _____	8. _____ _____ _____
9. (fill in) _____ _____ _____	9. _____ _____ _____

easier to quit smoking if you have developed a program of physical activity that enables you to use exercise to help suppress and replace smoking urges. Experience in bringing about beneficial change in stress management and in exercise habits will not only equip you with specific skills useful in breaking the smoking habit but will also give you increased confidence that you *can* quit.

TWO: BUILDING COMMITMENT
TO QUIT SMOKING

As mentioned in earlier chapters, success in any attempt at self-directed change requires a major initial effort, followed by a gradual decrease in conscious effort as new life-styles become more automatic. To augment your commitment, write a self-contract in which you state your intention to quit smoking. Follow the total plan described in this chapter rather than selecting out small pieces. There are clearly options and places for personal experimenting, but innovations should be placed within a carefully planned total program.

At times, turmoil in your personal life may make it difficult to carry through with your plans. Rather than embarking on a program during a particularly hectic period, I strongly recommend that you delay beginning your effort until you have a two- to three-week period of relatively stable social and work schedules that allows you to give your program an optimal chance to succeed.

It will be helpful to gain the social support of at least one other person, preferably an ex-smoker. (Your local chapter of the American Cancer Society can furnish you with names of ex-smokers who have volunteered to work with would-be ex-smokers.) This buddy-system approach has been found to be particularly effective. An alternative method is to assemble a group of ex-smokers to furnish social support. Make a statement to these persons (for instance, through the self-contract method) that you are going to quit. This step gives your decision greater commitment, and your friends can participate by encouraging you and checking on your progress. Family members or co-workers will be better able to help if they become familiar with the principles of self-directed change and work with you, or on their own, on some of the change programs contained in this book.

THREE: INCREASING AWARENESS OF
YOUR SMOKING PATTERNS

You have achieved the first level of awareness when you know how many cigarettes you smoke and your smoking-related cardiovascular risk. The second level of awareness is to gauge how strongly you desire each cigarette you smoke. The third level is to become aware of the circumstances or cues that trigger your smoking urges (finishing a meal, feeling tense, driving, drinking, etc.). You can monitor all three levels by keeping a smoking diary, recorded in a small spiral notebook or on a card inserted in the cigarette pack. An example of such a diary is on the next page.

You can be flexible in creating a diary that works effectively for you. The diary shown here is only one of many that can be used successfully. Many smokers find that simplified recording methods work satisfactorily. The important point is that you learn what cues trigger your desire to smoke and which carry the strongest urge. During the first week of recording, train yourself to increase your sensitivity to the strength of your smoking urges or cravings (later in this chapter you will focus on ways to suppress these urges). Every cigarette is preceded by an urge that can be rated, though some low-urge smoking is almost automatic. You can refine your diary by noting the times when you have an urge to smoke and yet do not (e.g., by circling the rating number of 1, 2, 3, or 4 in your diary only for the urges that are actually followed by smoking).

During the second week of your record keeping, focus on identifying the cues that precede your desire to smoke. It is useful to know, for example, whether or not you show a strong tendency to smoke in response to stress and tension. If you do, the stress reduction methods (which are useful for *all* categories of smoking) will be particularly important to you. In addition to the cues mentioned in the sample diary, think of other circumstances that may trigger your desire to smoke. These might include: (1) when you wake up; (2) when the telephone rings; (3) when you are angry; (4) when you are happy; (5) when you smell cigarette smoke; (6) or when you are in the smoking section of a plane or restaurant. Smoking urges can be precipitated either by external circumstances or by internal mental events.

FOUR: BUILDING AN ACTION PLAN
FOR SUCCESSFUL QUITTING

You are now ready to develop an action plan to quit smoking. The sequence and methods recommended here are ones considered best for a self-help format. Most studies of methods for quitting have involved face-to-face contact with instructors or therapists. However, the Stanford Center for Research in Disease Prevention has

SAMPLE DIARY OF SMOKING TIMES, CUES, AND URGES

Date _____

Time	Cue	Urge	Time	Cue	Urge
7:00 A.M.	M, C	4, 3	4:00 P.M.		
8:00	D, D, T	2, 2, 1	5:00	D, D, D	1, 1, 1
9:00			6:00	A, A	3, 1
10:00	C	2	7:00	M	4
11:00	T, U	3, 1	8:00		
12:00 NOON	M	4	9:00	T	4
1:00 P.M.			10:00	A, A, S	2, 1, 1
2:00	T, B, T	1, 2, 1	11:00		
3:00	S	1	12:00 MIDNIGHT		

Total number cigarettes smoked = 23

Key:
M = After meals
D = Driving
T = Tense or under time pressure
C = Drinking coffee
S = Social reminder, (e.g., seeing
    another smoker)
A = Drinking alcohol
B = Bored
U = Uncertain or unknown

Rating of Intensity of Urge:
Scale of 1 through 4, with 4 indicating
the strongest desire

achieved successful results with methods that focus on the individual's capacity to achieve desired changes on his or her own, given the proper tools.

The major skills needed to quit smoking have been described in Chapters 3 and 4. These skills, plus a few additional ones, will be described under three categories: (1) tapering, (2) quitting, and (3) maintenance.

Tapering

Almost all confirmed smokers who have experienced major difficulties in stopping are persons who smoke more than 15 cigarettes a day. If you are in this group of smokers, your objective during a tapering period is to bring your daily smoking rate down to a level of 12 to 15 cigarettes a day. Cutting your daily rate *below* that level is more difficult and also carries with it the danger that each cigarette you do smoke will be strongly desired and thus more rewarding. Tapering to the 12-15 cigarette level before quitting entirely allows you to learn how to suppress your urge to smoke, as well as to learn other skills that are helpful when you finally quit smoking entirely.

(If you currently smoke about 12 cigarettes per day, you can reduce your rate to about 8 or 9 during this period.) Practice to gain proficiency in the skills used during the tapering phase as they will also be needed in the quitting and maintenance stages. These skills are (1) suppressing the urge to smoke, (2) activating social support, and (3) developing alternatives incompatible with smoking.

Suppressing the Urge to Smoke. The method described in the following drill, if well developed, can be a mainstay of your quitting program since it equips you to attack your problem at its source—the craving for another cigarette. This urge suppression method, which

---

SMOKING URGE SUPPRESSION DRILL

1. When you feel a definite craving for a cigarette, allow your mind to focus on the craving.

2. Think of a negative image of the effects of smoking on your body (e.g., you feel hot and scratchy air going in and out of your lungs; you are inside your lungs and, as a Lilliputian, are looking at a honeycomb that has been dipped in dirty motor oil; you are exhaling an unpleasant odor and people are turning away from you; your skin is becoming wrinkled and aged as the nicotine and carbon monoxide circulate in your body; your arteries are becoming clogged with deposits of fatty scar tissue).

3. Wait until you feel the unpleasantness of the negative imagery. At this point your urge, desire, or craving for a cigarette should be reduced or abolished.

4. Now start a self-reward sequence, beginning with a relaxation drill. If you are a skilled relaxer, you can achieve rather complete deep muscle and mental relaxation within a few minutes. You should now notice further reduction in any residual urge to smoke.

5. Complete the pleasant state of relaxation with a positive image as a further reward for your success in suppressing your urge to smoke. The image can be anything pleasant, or it can be linked to the specific potential benefits of successfully quitting smoking (e.g., you are looking at a peaceful, blue mountain stream; you feel clean fresh air flowing through your lungs; you are a Lilliputian inside your lungs looking at a honeycomb structure that is pink and healthy; your breath is pleasant and you are now more attractive to others; your sense of taste and smell are returning; you feel relaxed and full of energy).

---

relies on imagery and relaxation skills already familiar to you from practice in Chapter 4, can be invoked at the first sign of an urge to smoke. (The earlier the chain of behavior leading to smoking can be broken, the greater your chance of success.) Your ability to suppress smoking urges will increase with practice. Before you begin, brush up on your imagery and relaxation skills (see Chapter 4).

Think of both positive and negative images of your own; practice them until you find the ones that work best for you. The most important test is that you can actually *see* and *feel* the images and emotions that you wish to evoke.

You can practice short, intermediate, and long versions of the Urge Suppression Drill. As you develop skill, you will be able to run through a successful sequence within as short a time as a minute (in doing so you will engage in very brief flashes of negative images, shift to an Instant Relaxation Drill, then evoke a brief positive image). Be sure to allow adequate time during each phase to develop the feelings and images. You might use longer periods of imagery and relaxation to suppress the stronger urges you encounter. But in order to use urge suppression practically (e.g., during work, social occasions, or driving) you will need to develop enough skill so that you can do an Urge Suppression Drill almost instantly, and as often as necessary.

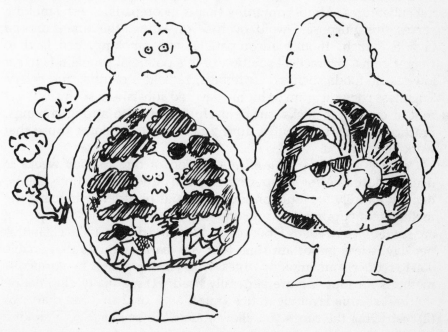

Activating Social Support. Enlist social support from a variety of sources. If you have identified an ex-smoker friend, engage his or her help during your tapering period in a manner that is convenient for both of you (e.g., a phone call every few days to provide general encouragement). Another form of support is available from family, friends, and co-workers. Bring them into your plans, ask them to help bolster your effort, and tell them that you will be announcing the date you are going to quit within the next month, assuming that your tapering program goes smoothly.

Developing Smoking Substitutes. The use of deep muscle relaxation as part of the urge suppression method has been described; practicing deep muscle and mental relaxation alone can also be quite successful in suppressing smoking urges. Another alternative—engaging in physical activity—is also effective in countering smoking urges. Exercise can range from brief walks to more vigorous types of preplanned activity. Although exercise breaks are useful as immediate smoking substitutes when taken soon after you feel an urge to smoke, a routine of vigorous physical exercise, engaged in three to four times a week, very likely carries with it more prolonged benefits—reducing both the strength and frequency of cravings. (There may be psychological as well as physical reasons for reduced nicotine craving after vigorous exercise.)

In addition to relaxation and exercise, you can devise other smoking substitutes. Almost anything that is incompatible with smoking serves this purpose. Avoid overuse of eating, the time-honored favorite which, though incompatible with smoking, can lead to weight gains. A practical solution to this potential problem is to eat low-calorie foods such as cucumbers, radishes, carrots, and celery. Sugarless chewing gum or highly flavored substances such as ginger root or cinnamon sticks can be useful counters to strong cravings. Practice various substitutes during tapering to discover those that work best for you.

Devising a Tapering Schedule. A period of one to four weeks is usually desirable for a tapering effort. The length of time should depend entirely on your confidence in your proficiency in using the methods for suppressing smoking urges; longer periods of tapering are sometimes needed. How you reduce smoking to 12-15 cigarettes per day is less important than that you learn methods that enable you to reduce your smoking urges while cutting down. Two principal methods for tapering are generally used: (1) gradually eliminating the lowest-urge-level cigarettes (rated as 1 or 2 in your diary) or (2) restricting the times you allow yourself to smoke (e.g., smoking once an hour on the hour). You might also gradually lengthen the intervals between smoking (e.g., through the use of pocket timers). I find the first method preferable since it alerts you to your smoking urges.

Sometime during your tapering period, set a date when you will quit smoking; announce this date to your social support group. You may gain extra incentive if the quitting date has a special significance for you (New Year's Day, a birthday, the first day of spring, etc.).

Creating a Tapering Period Self-Contract. Given the complexity of your plans for the tapering period, a self-contract can help clarify your goals. See the example below.

SELF-CONTRACT FOR AN ACTION PLAN FOR TAPERING

Date: _____

To taper my smoking, I will enlist the aid of _____. I plan to reduce smoking from an average of 24 cigarettes a day to 15 a day over a three-week period by cutting down on cigarettes in my lowest-urge category (particularly those smoked while driving or when I am tense or bored). I will use an Urge Suppression Drill at least three times a day in response to smoking urges and will exercise vigorously (e.g., jog, swim, etc.) at least three times a week as a general antidote to my desire to smoke.

My responsibilities are to record daily the number of cigarettes I smoke, the number of times I use an Urge Suppression Drill or a short walk to decrease my urge to smoke (and to rate their effectiveness), and to record the number of times a week I exercise vigorously.

My helper's responsibilities are to telephone me every three days for general encouragement and to inquire about my progress.

Our joint responsibilities are to meet in one week to review my progress. At that time I will announce the date I have chosen to quit smoking.

Date: _____ Signed: _____
Review date: _____ Helper: _____

Scheduled Smoking Week

A week before your intended quitting date, begin a "scheduled smoking week"; during this week smoke *only four* cigarettes a day—

and at a rate close to or slightly faster than your usual rate. (You should be proficient by now in magnifying through imagery the negative effects of smoking.) Schedule a time to smoke your first cigarette; immediately after finishing it, smoke a second cigarette just as you did the first. Schedule your smoking of the two remaining cigarettes at least an hour later. You should be able to finish smoking two cigarettes in this manner in about 15 minutes. Do this every day for seven days.

Figure 8-1 depicts the time sequences and an example of daily cigarette smoking during the smoking-cessation stages described in this chapter.

Time your regular smoking rate; most people take a puff about every 25 seconds. Speed this up to one puff every 15 or 20 seconds during scheduled smoking. (Do not smoke more rapidly than that since it can be harmful.) You should be reasonably free of distractions during these 15-minute sessions. The purpose of scheduled smoking is to imprint vividly on your mind and body the *unpleasant* aspects of smoking. This will work only if you have been able to

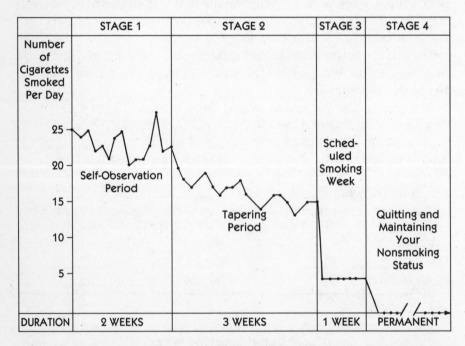

Figure 8-1: Examples of smoking rates for an average smoker during the four stages of smoking cessation. (The tapering period may be of variable length.)

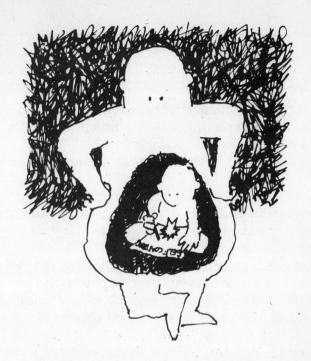

achieve some success in using the negative imagery practiced in your Urge Suppression Drill during the tapering period.

During the scheduled smoking week, be sure to smoke the allotted cigarettes at preplanned times, preferably when you do not feel an urge to smoke. Focus on the hot, scratchy feeling of the smoke going through your throat and into your lungs. Blow smoke into your hand and back into your face. Concentrate on the sensation of your throat feeling sore and raw. Devise other negative images of your own that evoke unpleasant aspects of smoking. Many ex-smokers report that the feeling of nausea is readily evoked and revived in later practice without smoking. Your exposure during this scheduled smoking week to 14 *unpleasant* experiences associated with smoking can help you maintain a nonsmoking status once you quit.

Carry out your scheduled smoking using the following drill. Practice this drill twice a day (with at least one hour between sessions) for seven days prior to your final quitting day.

It is critical that you smoke no more than four cigarettes per day during your scheduled smoking week. If you do not stick to your plan, you become highly vulnerable to relapse. If you find yourself

SCHEDULED SMOKING DRILL

Practice this drill at a time when you do not feel much desire to smoke.

1. Sit or recline in a comfortable setting.

2. Practice a relaxation drill for a few minutes. Develop a feeling that you can easily do without a smoke.

3. Light your first cigarette and take a puff about every 15-20 seconds.

4. Concentrate on each puff and imagine hot, scratchy smoke going through your throat into your lungs. Pay attention to and magnify any unpleasant sensation. Imagine that your throat is dry and sore from smoking.

5. Imagine other negative aspects of smoking, derived from the negative images you used in your Urge Suppression Drill.

6. Light your second cigarette as soon as you finish your first. Continue to feel and imagine unpleasant aspects of smoking this cigarette.

7. Focus on the negative feelings you experienced for at least five minutes after finishing your second cigarette.

8. Record in your diary the degree of unpleasantness you felt on a rating from 0 to 4, with 4 being most unpleasant.

---

unable to maintain this four-cigarette-per-day rate, return to the tapering stage and reexamine your smoking patterns. You have many options. For example, you could remain at the tapering stage of 12-15 cigarettes per day for a few more weeks, during which time you would continue to practice the Urge Suppression Drill, exercise, and attain further skill in stress management. Do not allow a return to an earlier stage to destroy your morale. Use this period to refuel your commitment, strengthen your social support network, and increase your skill in suppressing your smoking urges.

You will need to employ a variety of techniques to suppress your smoking urges during the scheduled smoking week. Your most valuable tool will be the Urge Suppression Drill; use it when urges develop, and as often as needed. In addition, actively involve your social support team during this critical week (e.g., through daily telephone calls or face-to-face contact). Extra periods of deep muscle relaxation and increased use of vigorous physical activity will also be helpful. (In our studies at Stanford we have yet to find a serious adult runner who smokes, although a few beginning joggers still do so.)

Some people need special incentives to get through the scheduled smoking week. You can obtain such incentives by using a self-contract in which a designated sum of money, for example, is temporarily transferred to your buddy or to an intermediary with the agreement that the money will go to a charity if you do not follow your plan.

Use of Nicotine-Containing Chewing Gum

A new method has appeared that may double your chances of successful quitting. This method entails use of sticks of gum containing either 2 or 4 mg of nicotine in a slowly released form, sold as *Nicorette*. When chewed for 30 minutes the nicotine enters the blood stream and produces blood levels of nicotine adequate to relieve some of the cravings for a cigarette. The gum is prescribed by physicians and is best used 4 to 6 times a day for 2 to 6 months after quitting. For first-time quit attempts it is advisable to do so without the help of the gum. If the gum is used, the time to start it is during the scheduled smoking week but only as a sampling experience on 3 or 4 occasions to get used to the experience. All use should await directions from your physician to begin on your quitting day. It is critically important to use all of these self-help methods along with the gum. Using gum alone is really no better than a simple "cold-turkey" approach.

Quitting Day

After successfully completing your scheduled smoking week, you are ready to quit. On your quitting day and thereafter, you will be calling upon the same techniques you used during scheduled smoking to suppress your smoking urges—the Urge Suppression Drill, relaxation techniques, vigorous physical exercise, and your social support network.

FIVE: EVALUATING YOUR SMOKING CESSATION PROGRAM

Throughout your action plan to quit smoking, you will be evaluating the effectiveness of your efforts and the skills that you have developed. Check the records you have been keeping to see how well you are achieving your goals and to detect problem areas that need special attention (e.g., smoking urges arising in stressful situations at work, social gatherings, etc.). You now have the skills to devise your own plan to suppress particularly persistent smoking urges.

Rebuild your commitment at intervals throughout your program when you find yourself becoming discouraged. Do this by listing the positive aspects of your effort to quit—think of small successes and unexpected benefits (e.g., you feel healthier, you have more energy, etc.). Again, it is important not to be overly harsh or critical of your efforts; smoking is an especially difficult habit to break and it takes practice to feel fully comfortable as a nonsmoker.

SIX: MAINTENANCE

Once you have quit, your goal is to become increasingly comfortable with being a nonsmoker. To do this, maintain and increase your proficiency in the various methods you used to decrease smoking urges. Continue to use the Urge Suppression Drill and relaxation drills regularly. Also, continue to use exercise as a way to decrease smoking urges. Be inventive in devising ways to maintain the involvement and social support of your friends and family.

To consolidate your nonsmoking skills, practice behavioral rehearsal (see Chapter 4). Pay special attention to self-reward. Behavioral rehearsal can help you resist a potential relapse by teaching you how to strengthen your mental defenses against smoking urges, how to turn down a persuasive offer of a cigarette, how to handle your withdrawal symptoms, and how to feel comfortable being a nonsmoker.

The first behavioral rehearsal method is a modified Urge Suppression Drill, following the sequence of focusing on (1) the urge to smoke, (2) a negative image, (3) relaxation, (4) a positive image. The modification is that you create the urge to smoke within your imagination rather than waiting for the urges to occur naturally. This method will give you the opportunity to practice urge suppression at times of your own choosing and thus increase your proficiency.

A second type of behavioral rehearsal is also useful. It is a role-playing exercise that can be done alone or with the assistance of a friend or family member (preferably an ex-smoker). There are two roles: the person trying to persuade you to smoke and the person trying to resist. If you do the drill alone, you can play both roles, first persuader, then resister.

What follows is a sample script. After reading it, devise your own drill. You may encounter persuasive arguments to resume smoking

SAMPLE BEHAVIORAL REHEARSAL DRILL FOR EX-SMOKERS

Arguments to Smoke	Arguments to Remain a Nonsmoker
1. Come on, one cigarette won't hurt.	1. No thanks. I don't want one; I worked hard to quit and I'm glad that I have.
2. Keep me company, join me in a smoke.	2. I'll keep you company but I don't smoke anymore. Why don't you try quitting and keep *me* company?
3. You're so irritable, you need a cigarette. You're too jumpy these days.	3. That wouldn't do me any good. My body is still adjusting to going without nicotine. Encourage me in my effort to quit. I'll exercise to get rid of my nervous energy.
4. Aren't you afraid of gaining weight? Smoking sure keeps my weight down; I just balloon up when I stop smoking.	4. I'm not afraid of gaining weight, because I'm not allowing myself to eat more. I'm also exercising more, which cuts down on my appetite and my smoking urges, too.
5. How can you quit after so many years—wouldn't you rather just keep smoking?	5. It feels great to have kicked the habit after all these years. I feel better and happier, and I have a sense of accomplishment.
6. Try this new filter cigarette. It's really rated low in tar and nicotine. You don't need to worry about smoking if you use these.	6. If I get used to smoking again, I might get hooked on cigarettes higher in tar and nicotine. Besides, heart attacks and strokes are caused by the carbon monoxide levels of cigarette smoke as well as by nicotine and tar. It's not worth it to quit halfway; I prefer being a nonsmoker.
7. The silent offer—the outstretched pack.	7. I'd appreciate it if you would not offer me cigarettes anymore.
8. Come on, you're going to die sooner or later anyway.	8. I'd prefer later than sooner. Incidentally, smoking may increase the aging process; it may encourage wrinkling of the skin.

(coming from within yourself or from others), and behavioral rehearsal can help give you a sudden reflex defense for unguarded moments of stress, tension, or discouragement that could otherwise trigger a return to smoking.

Take the time to develop your own drill, since practice with concepts you generate is by far the most valuable. It is up to you when, where, and how often you use the role-playing method of behavioral rehearsal. I suggest that you plan a maintenance program that is quite intensive for the first few weeks. As you become more skillful at suppressing your desire to smoke, you will become progressively more comfortable in being a nonsmoker.

Booster Sessions

Booster sessions using the two behavioral rehearsal drills are helpful if you feel your smoking urges are returning in a stronger form or if for any reason you feel tempted to resume smoking. Such symptoms are an early warning sign that you need to strengthen your urge suppression skills. Also enlist additional help and encouragement from your social support group. Once you quit, it is important to avoid having that first cigarette. Hence, a return to scheduled smoking, coupled with negative imagery, should *not* be used unless you have a smoking relapse. If you do experience a minor relapse, be careful not to label yourself a failure—that will unleash negative thoughts that are detrimental to achieving lasting changes. Feelings of failure are invitations to give up and throw away all that has been learned and accomplished. Quickly return to your nonsmoking state if you do have a few cigarettes. To innoculate yourself against harmful, self-defeatist thinking if you resume your previous smoking level, follow these steps in which you reiterate to yourself that you can *quickly* regain your nonsmoking status:

1. Calmly accept that your return to a full rate of smoking indicates that smoking is still residually attractive to you and that smoking exerted its power over you through that attractiveness.

2. Taper again to 12-15 cigarettes and follow with your rapid smoking week and evaluation and maintenance programs, as you did before. Do this in a matter-of-fact way with the simple and practical goal of imprinting on your mind and body that smoking is unpleasant and therefore unattractive. You may have had years of dealing with cigarettes as attractive and perhaps only a few weeks or months to create your new set of responses. Do not be discouraged. Use booster sessions to augment your skills and enlist support from

your friends. Consider addition of the nicotine-containing gum on your second try.

Special Problems

Weight Gain. The average weight gained by ex-smokers is about three pounds—and even that is usually transient. Weight gains can be readily countered. Avoid snacking between meals to suppress smoking urges; if you do snack, eat low-calorie foods. Refer to Chapter 7 for other ways to avoid weight gains. There is no reason to be unduly concerned or worried about gaining weight. You can use effective relaxation methods or exercise to handle the problem. These methods will decrease the desire for food and, in the case of exercise, will decrease body weight as well.

Withdrawal Symptoms. You will usually have symptoms related to the withdrawal of your body from its dependency on nicotine, which causes a true physical addiction. These symptoms commonly take the form of lethargy or irritability. Do not be alarmed; both will disappear with time and both are partly relieved by exercise or relaxation. Forewarned is forearmed. It is these symptoms that the nicotine gum will relieve while you deal with the many psychological addictions to smoking that you acquired.

Initial Failure. Some people may not succeed in their initial efforts to quit. If you still have trouble after your first few tries, the following steps will help keep you moving in the right direction: (1) Temporarily seek to lower your cardiovascular risk in another area first and later return to your program to quit smoking. (2) Continue to smoke the smallest number of cigarettes that you can tolerate—perhaps this will be the 12-15 a day of the tapering period. (3) Change to filtered cigarettes to reduce your nicotine and tar exposure, but remember that the carbon monoxide of cigarette smoke (which is the factor responsible for atherosclerosis) remains high even in filter cigarettes. Pipes or cigars, or cigarette smoking without inhaling, are interim alternatives that cut risk considerably. However, cigarette smokers must be particularly careful not to inhale their pipe or cigar smoke unwittingly. If drinking makes you want to smoke or contributes to your difficulty in quitting, decrease your alcohol intake before you attempt to quit smoking again. (Skill in stress management will enable you to suppress your desire for alcohol as well as for cigarettes.)

Although it is not easy to quit smoking and success will not occur overnight, even the confirmed chain-smoker can quit. It is worth the effort.

9 WHERE DO WE GO FROM HERE?

One day in 1952, as a medical student in San Francisco, I had an experience that was to become a powerful influence in my life. I was assigned a patient, Mr. W.D., a 38-year-old salesman from Sacramento, California, who had just had a severe heart attack. After a stormy course he recovered, and I continued to care for him while I was an intern and later a resident. During this time and following his death four years later, I learned that neither I nor the medical care system as a whole knew what to do for Bill; I saw him and others like him who had taken their well-being for granted yearn for health *after* a devastating and life-threatening event had wrenched it away. I experienced the bond of trust and affection that can occur between the physician and the family unit in which the patient lives. I felt the deep grief of a family that follows the disability and premature loss of one of its members—a grief that belies the glib notion that a heart attack or a stroke is "a nice clean way to go." Both Bill and my friend Roger, who died 25 years later, were considered to be "healthy," vital men. Their deaths left their families with the stunning frustration that inevitably follows such a senseless, preventable loss.

My relationship with Bill and his family was my first close encounter with coronary heart disease. In the years since I met Bill, the medical profession has acquired vast knowledge about heart disease, yet we are still watching the epidemic of premature heart attack and stroke sweep through the world at varying rates of ascent and descent. We also see huge differences among the world's peoples in rates of various cancers and diabetes and we know that diet and obesity are heavily involved. Often, when viewing the advances of medicine, I think of the words of Herodotus: "Of all man's miseries, the bitterest is this, to know so much and to have control over nothing."

Today I ask both myself and you, *Where do we go from here?* Can we use the storehouse of medical knowledge and wisdom we have gained since the time of Herodotus to influence our destiny? Clearly we *can*. At a personal level, the previous chapters have provided methods of self-directed change that can assist you and your family to live fuller, healthier lives and to greatly lower your risk of developing cardiovascular disease and, very likely, some forms of cancer, as well as diabetes and osteoporosis.

Beyond the personal level, where do we go from here? If you and your family make needed changes to alter hazardous health habits, will those changes be positively reinforced by the larger social forces around you? Will the foods you and your family want to eat be readily available in restaurants or in school cafeterias? If you teach your children to eat healthy, whole, natural foods and not to smoke, will they be able to resist the unhealthy influences they will inevitably encounter? Will they gain more power in their lives to resist peer pressures to use drugs or alcohol? Will your own resolve to exercise or to manage stress more effectively be aided or countered by your environment?

We cannot ignore the larger social forces that promote and maintain ill health in the prevailing popular culture. Otherwise, we find ourselves in the frustrating predicament of the aprocryphal man who is so busy rescuing drowning people floating by his narrow field of vision that he gives no thought to, and has no control over, the upstream forces that are creating the havoc in the first place. It is truly absurd for the medical care apparatus in our country to wait until people are sick, chronically ill, or disabled to be concerned about their health.

How can we develop "upstream" societal changes to complement and augment our individual efforts? First, by adopting healthier habits, we can in fact help set in motion a change in others through the beneficial effects of our own example and the sharing of our experiences with others. Our personal food-buying habits can provide an economic incentive for food suppliers to increase the availability of healthy, unadulterated foods. Our nation is ready for consumer pressure to extend to such issues as cigarette advertising in magazines and newspapers and promotion of products like chewing tobacco at sports events.

Second, by becoming involved in local community affairs, we can further accelerate change toward healthier life-styles. Elementary and high schools need the ongoing interest of knowledgeable citizens to insure that school lunches are nutritious and that the curriculum includes high quality health education and physical education. Adult health classes can be developed by local school districts and community colleges. If our children are taught self-directed change methods in these classes they can gain ability to resist peer pressure to adopt drugs and alcohol as well as cigarettes or fast foods. Businesses can provide training in stress management and nutrition and can provide facilities and incentives for employees to exercise. As citizens we can make our voices heard in city and county governments to bring about expansion of recreational areas, bicycle paths, and parks. We can also give much needed support to volunteer health associations such as the American Heart Association, the American Cancer Society, and the American Lung Association.

A third avenue for bringing about needed societal change is in the arena of national policy. Let me mention a few changes that could help reinforce our personal and community efforts: (1) The U.S. Public Health Service and state health departments should continue to expand their present involvement in health education to share with the public recently acquired medical knowledge. (2) The National Institutes of Health should further expand their growing support for research in health education, nutrition, and studies on how to organize communities most effectively to achieve self-help at low cost. (3) Private research foundations should join in a major role in prevention, as the Kaiser Family Foundation, the Carnegie Foundation, and the Kellog Foundation have done. (4) Schools for health professionals (including schools of medicine, public health, nursing, and dentistry) should increase their adult education programs, as well as their faculties, in nutrition and preventive medicine. (5) The Food and Drug Administration should move beyond its current preoccupation with chemical additives to consider the role of salt, sugar, saturated fat, and cholesterol in chronic disease causation. (6) Unemployment and lack of meaningful work create a vicious circle of despair and ill health for millions of our citizens; surely American ingenuity and our tradition of fairness can produce imaginative policies that help rather than blame the victim. (7) Multiple citizens' lobbies should be organized to inform the public on health issues and to influence state and national legislation on these issues.

Spiraling health costs downstream will increasingly force us to look upstream in order to bridge the glaring gap between resources allocated to repair and those allocated to prevention. In order to reduce chronic illness, disability, and death resulting from avoidable environmental hazards, more resources must be channeled into preventive medicine. This will happen only when the public manifests this demand through the political process. The time has come for us to act both separately as individuals and together as a nation to heal ourselves.

READER'S GUIDE

n giving talks on prevention of chronic diseases to laymen and professionals, I have found that many more questions are raised than can be answered. So it will be, and appropriately so, with this book. Hence, this section will direct you to a variety of sources for further exploration of the subjects I have discussed. Books, magazines, technical articles, and various organizations are listed under the relevant chapter headings.

CHAPTERS 1 AND 2

An excellent scholarly discussion of cardiovascular risk factors is presented by Drs. Henry Blackburn and Russell Luepker in "Heart Disease," *Public Health and Preventive Medicine*, 12th ed., ed. by John Last (New York: Appleton-Century-Crofts, 1985). A general philosophy of preventive medicine is described in "The Responsibility of the Individual," by John Knowles, in *Doing Better and Feeling Worse: Health in the United States*, ed. by John Knowles (New York: W.W. Norton, 1977), and *Man Adapting* by René Dubos (New Haven: Yale University Press, 1965). *Who Shall Live?* by Victor Fuchs (New York: Basic Books, 1975) and *America's Health Care Revolution* by Joseph Califano, Jr. (New York: Random House, 1986) are incisive books on the economics of health care. *Vitality and Aging* by Drs. James Fries and Lawrence Crapo (New York: W. H. Freeman, 1981) is also a very useful book, particularly in setting a theoretical foundation for the primacy of decreasing illness rather than merely increasing life span.

Technical journals that can keep you abreast of new developments in the causes and prevention of chronic diseases such as cancer, cardiovascular disease, and diabetes include *The New England Journal of Medicine* (10 Shattuck St., Boston, MA 02115), *The Journal of the American Medical Association* (535 N. Dearborn St., Chicago, IL 60610), *American Journal of Epidemiology* (624 N. Broadway, Rm. 225, Baltimore, MD 21205), and *Preventive Medicine* (Academic Press, Inc., P.O. Box 6550, Duluth, MN 55806).

CHAPTER 3

Prior to embarking on self-directed change, the subject of this chapter, it is often necessary to determine whether a problem exists that may need medical care. A very useful book for this purpose is *Take Care of Yourself: A Consumer's Guide to Medical Care* by Donald M. Vickery and James Fries (Reading, MA: Addison-Wesley, 1981). *How People Change* by Allen Wheelis (New York: Harper and Row, 1974) and *I Can If I Want To* by Arnold Lazarus and Allen Fay (New York: Warner Books, 1977) are practical books that may be useful in augmenting self-directed change efforts. More technical books providing an important background of psychological theories underlying self-directed change techniques include the following: *Theories of Learning*, 4th ed. by Gordon Bower and Ernest Hilgard (Englewood Cliffs, NJ: Prentice-Hall, 1981); and *Social Learning Theory* by Albert Bandura (Englewood Cliffs, NJ: Prentice-Hall, 1977). The book by Kathryn and Michael Mahoney discussed in this chapter, *Permanent Weight Control*, is available from W. W. Norton (New York).

Technical journals that deal with research concerning self-directed change include *The Journal of Behavioral Medicine* (Plenum Press, 233 Spring St., New York, NY 10013), *The Journal of Consulting and Clinical Psychology* (1200 17th St. NW, Washington, DC 20036), and *Cognitive Therapy and Research* (Plenum Press, 233 Spring St., New York, NY 10013). Given the importance of self-observation and recording techniques, you may wish to obtain a wrist-counter. A mechanical wrist-counter (worn like a wristwatch), each number being advanced by pressing a plunger, is a useful device as are various types of bead-counters. Choose a wrist-counter that will allow you to do separate counting of more than one type of item (e.g., two rows could be used for counting the number of smoking urges experienced and two for counting the number of times you smoke).

CHAPTER 4

The following books are well-suited for extending your stress management skills: *Put Your Mother on the Ceiling: Children's Imagination Games* by Richard DeMille (Santa Barbara, CA: Santa Barbara Press, 1981). *Learn to Relax: 13 Ways to Reduce Tension* by C. Eugene Walker (Englewood Cliffs, NJ: Prentice-Hall, 1975); *Beyond the Relaxation Response* by Herbert Benson and William Proctor (New York: Berkley Publishing Group, 1985), and *Stress and the Art of Biofeedback* by Barbara Brown (New York: Harper and Row, 1977) furnish a broad view of the subject of biofeedback. A technical article of excellent breadth that reviews the relationship between stress and coronary disease is "Psychological and Social Risk Factors for Coronary Disease," Parts 1 and 2, by Dr. C. David Jenkins (*New England Journal of Medicine*, vol. 294, nos. 18 and 19, 1976, pp. 987-94 and 1033-38). Reprints of this article are available from the Department of Psychiatry, University of Texas, 301 University Blvd., Galveston, TX 77550.

CHAPTER 5

Walking My Way by John Merrill (Topsfield, MA, c/o Merrimack Publishers' Circle; Chatto & Windus, The Hogarth Press, 1984) and Gary Yanker's *The Complete Book of Exercise Walking* (Chicago: Contemporary Books, 1983) contain good suggestions on safe walking and inspire the reader to practice this basic form of locomotion more often. For people interested in the more strenuous exercise of mountain hiking, a definitive guide is *The Complete Walker* by Colin Fletcher (New York: Alfred A. Knopf, 1986). The new periodical *The Walking Magazine* (Raben Publishing, 711 Boylston St., Boston, MA 02116) covers all aspects of walking as a basic form of exercise.

Aerobics (New York: M. Evans, 1968), *Total Well Being: The Complete Aerobics Program for Radiant Health Through Exercise and Diet* (New York: M. Evans, 1982), and *The New Aerobics* (New York: M. Evans, 1985) by Kenneth Cooper, are the landmark books on aerobics. Dr. Cooper's extensive charts, setting forth his aerobic point system, provide helpful guides to equivalent amounts of aerobic exercise obtainable through various types of physical activity. These books also suggest optimal exercise levels for various activities suited to men and women at different ages. *Run to Health* by Peter D. Wood (New York: Grosset and Dunlap, 1980) contains an authoritative and eloquent account of the medical issues related to running. *Bicycling Science* by Frank R. Whitt and David G. Wilson (Cambridge: MIT

Press, 1985) contains good advice on bicycling safely and motivates the reader to bicycle. Drs. Paul Milvy, W.F. Forbes, and K.S. Brown present a discussion of research indicating that exercise is of preventive value in "A Critical Review of Epidemiologic Studies of Physical Activity" (*Annals of the New York Academy of Sciences*, vol. 301, 1977, pp. 519-49). *The Physician and Sportsmedicine* (McGraw-Hill, 4530 West 77th St., Minneapolis, MN 55435) is a periodical that deals with medical aspects of sports.

Runners' World (Rodale Press, 33 E. Minor St., Emmaus, PA 18049) provides medical advice as well as information on running events, running equipment, etc. Good publications for bicyclists are *Bicycling*, also by Rodale Press, and *Bicycle Guide* (Raben/Bicycle Guide Partners, 711 Bolyston St., Boston, MA 02116).

The President's Council on Physical Fitness and Sports (450 5th Street, NW, Washington, D.C. 20001) is a good source of information on physical well-being. The YMCA has a long history of providing exercise facilities and instruction in physical fitness; it remains an excellent local source for such services. In addition, many YMCA groups have programs and classes for the rehabilitation of coronary patients as well as general classes in nutrition, stress management, weight control, and smoking. Your local high school or community college physical education departments are also likely to be good sources of information on the availability of sport and recreational facilities. Organizations such as the Sierra Club offer information on hiking and bicycling opportunities. (Write to: Sierra Club, 530 Bush Street, San Francisco, CA 94108 for information and/or the address of the chapter nearest you.)

In Chapter 5, I recommended the use of a pedometer for determining the number of miles you walk a day. Pedometers are, however, delicate instruments and I suggest they not be worn while running. A sturdier pedometer than earlier models is now available from Accusplit, 2290A Ringwood Ave., San Jose, CA 95131 (1-800-538-9750). Recently many electronic digital sport watches have become available for a very reasonable price. These timepieces have many functions that can help you keep track of your walking and running and help make these activities more enjoyable.

CHAPTER 6

Cancer Today: Origins, Prevention, and Treatment by Leslie Roberts (Institute of Medicine: National Academy Press, 2101 Constitution

Ave., NW, Washington, DC 20418, 1984) is an excellent source book that covers the topic of nutrition and cancer prevention.

A varied selection of books is available on food and nutrition. These include *The New American Diet: The Lifetime Family Eating Plan for Good Health* by Sonja and William Connor (New York: Simon & Schuster, 1986) and *Healthy-Heart Cookbook* by Ellen B. Kwadler and Lillian A. Czech (New York: Van Nostrand Reinhold/CBI, 1984). The following cookbooks will serve you well in Phase I of the alternative food pattern: *American Heart Association Cookbook* (New York: Ballantine, 1986), *Eat to Your Heart's Content: The Low Cholesterol Gourmet Cookbook* by Gordon and Kay Heiss (New York: New American Library, 1979), *The Fat and Sodium Control Cookbook* by Alma Payne and Dorothy Callahan (Boston: Little, Brown, 1975) and *Don't Eat Your Heart Out Cookbook* by Joseph and Bernie Piscatella (New York: Workman Publishing, 1983). *Deliciously Simple* by Harriet Roth (New York: New American Library, 1986) contains recipes designed especially for low-salt intake; however, you can easily reduce the salt levels given for recipes in other cookbooks as well. Ideas for flavoring your low-salt cooking with herbs and spices are available in *The Joy of Cooking* by Irma Rombauer and Marion Becker (New York: Macmillan, 1986) and *Herb Cookery* by Alan Hooker (San Francisco: 101 Productions, 1971).

Three reference books for identifying the salt, cholesterol, or fat content of various foods are *Barbara Kraus' Complete Guide to Sodium* (New York: New American Library, 1986) and *The Barbara Kraus Cholesterol Counter* (New York: Putman Publishing Group, 1985), and *The Fat Counter Guide* by Ronald M. Deutsch (Palo Alto, CA: Bull Publishing, 1978).

Although you may wish to use the books that follow in Phase I, they are especially useful in Phases II and III; all contain excellent vegetarian recipes. Modify the recipes as needed to lower salt content and to avoid a high butterfat and cholesterol intake (from milk, cheese, and egg yolks). The new edition of *Diet for a Small Planet* by Frances Moore Lappé (New York: Ballantine, 1986) is a splendid book that not only provides recipes but also discusses how, by eating vegetarian dishes, we can fill our protein needs and help conserve energy resources. *Recipes for a Small Planet* by Ellen B. Ewald (New York: Ballantine, 1986) and *Great Meatless Meals* by Frances Moore Lappé and Ellen B. Ewald (New York: Ballantine, 1984) offer additional meatless recipes, as do *The Vegetarian Epicure* by Anna Thomas (New York: Vintage, 1978), *Wings of Life: Whole Vegetarian Cookery* by

Julie Jordan (Trumansdale, NY: Crossing Press, 1976), and *The New Laurel's Kitchen* by Laurel Robertson, Carol Flinders, and Bronwen Godfrey (Berkeley, CA: Ten Speed Press, 1986). An unusual book by Mollie Katzen, *The Enchanted Broccoli Forest* (Berkeley, CA: Ten Speed Press, 1982), is a source of many eggless and low fat recipes adapted from the cooking of various countries.

Many books have recently appeared on Mediterranean and Oriental cooking, such as *Mediterranean Vegetarian Cooking* by Colin Spencer (New York: Thorsons Publishing, 1986), *The Book of Tofu* by William Shurtleff and Akino Aoyagi (Berkeley, CA: Ten Speed Press, 1983), *Madhur Jaffrey's World of the East Vegetarian Cooking* (New York: Alfred A. Knopf, 1984) and many others. Remember to replace butter and other animal fats with vegetable oils and when recipes call for eggs, use the whites only.

A book that combines good suggestions on diet and exercise is *The California Diet and Exercise Plan* by Peter Wood (Los Angeles: Medallion Books, 1983). Two other good books are *Jane Brody's Nutrition Book* (New York: Bantam, 1987) and *Jane Brody's Good Food Book, Living the High Carbohydrate Way* (New York: W.W. Norton, 1985).

An important technical review of the role of saturated fat and cholesterol in causing atherosclerosis is provided by Dr. Henry Blackburn's chapter "Diet and Mass Hyperlipidemia, Public Health Considerations," in *Nutrition, Lipids and Coronary Heart Disease* edited by Robert Levy, Basil Rifkind, Barbara Dennis, and Nancy Ernst (New York: Raven Press, 1979).

CHAPTER 7

A number of self-help books on weight control have appeared recently. A valuable book using self-directed change methods is *Permanent Weight Control: A Total Solution to the Dieter's Dilemma* by Michael and Kathryn Mahoney (New York: W.W. Norton, 1985). The following books are also useful: *Act Thin, Stay Thin* by Richard Stuart (New York: Jove Publications, 1985) and *Habits, Not Diets: The Real Way to Weight Control* by J.M. Ferguson (Palo Alto, CA: Bull Publishing, 1976).

A special problem in weight and high blood pressure control is associated with excessive social drinking. The following books apply methods of self-directed change to this problem: *Just One More* by James L. Free (New York: National Council on Alcoholism, 1977) and *Prevention of Alcohol Abuse* by Peter M. Miller and Ted Nirenberg (New York: Plenum Press, 1984).

A technical review of overweight and its relationship to high blood pressure is found in "Overweight and Hypertension" by B.N. Chiang, L.V. Perlman, and F.H. Epstein (*Circulation*, vol. 39, no. 3, 1969, pp. 403-22).

The best known weight-control group is Weight Watchers. Nonprofit self-help groups include Overeaters Anonymous (P.O. Box 92870, Los Angeles, CA 90009).

CHAPTER 8

Surprisingly few books have been written that provide effective self-directed methods for quitting smoking. One helpful book that does is *Break the Smoking Habit: A Behavioral Program for Giving up Cigarettes* by O.F. Pomerleau and C.S. Pomerleau (Hartford, CT: Behavioral Medicine Press, 1984).

A Smoking Gun by Elizabeth Whelan (Philadelphia, PA: George F. Stickley Co., 1984) is an excellent book covering the details of the role of the tobacco industry in pressuring magazines to delete articles about smoking and health and influencing politicians in relation to public policy on smoking.

A good account of research on smoking and health is found in *The Smoking Epidemic: A Matter of Worldwide Concern: Proceedings of the 4th World Conference on Smoking and Health*, ed. by L.M. Ramstrom (Philadelphia, PA: Coronet Books, 1980).

The Office for Smoking and Health (5600 Fishers Ln., Park Blvd. Room 110, Rockville, MD 20857), which incorporates the National Clearinghouse for Smoking and Health, is another important source of information on smoking research and education.

CHAPTER 9

To keep up with general health information, various health magazines are helpful. In addition to those already mentioned, *Prevention* (Rodale Press, 33 East Minor St., Emmaus, PA 18049, phone: 215-967-5171); *American Health* (80 Fifth Ave., New York, NY 10011); *Health* (Portland Place, Boulder, CO 80302); and *Consumer Reports* (Family Media Inc., 3 Park Ave., New York 10016) are reliable sources of general health information (although *Consumer Reports* of course, is not concerned only with health issues). Among the most important potential resources of continuing health education are the adult education services sponsored by local school and community college districts. These organizations are responsive to public requests, and there is much room for expansion of existing programs.

Nonprofit health associations are another vital and important resource, and they can benefit both from your financial support and your efforts as a volunteer. The American Heart Association (national headquarters: 7320 Greenville Ave., Dallas, TX 75231) is the major volunteer health association in the United States. It plays a large and important role not only in supporting ongoing research into the causes and treatment of cardiovascular disease, but also in providing valuable education on the prevention of heart attack and stroke. Every state in the United States has a state branch of the Heart Association and most have local and county branches. A visit, call, or letter to your local branch will enable you to become informed about the range of services available in your area.

The American Cancer Society (90 Park Avenue, New York, NY 10017), another large and effective volunteer health organization, has become increasingly interested in cancer prevention and can, for example, supply you with names of ex-smokers who can help you if you embark on a smoking-cessation program. The American Lung Association (1740 Broadway, New York, NY 10019) is also involved in research and education for the prevention of smoking.

The following three clearinghouses on health topics can be very helpful:

1. The Center for Medical Consumers (237 Thompson Street, New York, NY 10012; phone 212-674-9105). They will assist you by mail or telephone and publish an excellent newsletter, *Health Facts*, twelve times a year.

2. The National Health Information Clearinghouse (P.O. Box 1133, Washington, DC 20013).

3. The Planetree Health Resource Center (2040 Webster Street, San Francisco, CA 94115, phone: 415-346-4636) covers medical issues as well as issues of chronic disease prevention.

Consumer organizations such as the Center for Science in the Public Interest (1501 16th Street, NW, Washington, DC 20036) and the Consumers Union (256 Washington St., Mt. Vernon, NY 10550), publisher of *Consumer Reports*, offer a means of letting your health concerns be heard. Another organization, Action for Children's Television (20 University Road, Cambridge, MA 02138), is a valuable source of information on food-related advertising directed at children.

The Office of Disease Prevention and Health Promotion of the Public Health Service (Dept. of Health and Human Services, 330 C Street, Washington, DC 20201) is an important clearinghouse for information on disease prevention activities in both the private and public sectors. The Center for Health Promotion and Education of the Centers for Disease Control (1600 Clifton Road NE, Atlanta, GA 30333) has expanded its activities on many fronts and is an excellent source for information.

The Kaiser Family Foundation, Menlo Park, CA 94025, has recently launched an ambitious national program for health promotion that will include public education and technical assistance to communities through establishment of health promotion resource centers. The first of the four proposed centers has been established at Stanford University (Health Promotion Resource Center, 1000 Welch Road, Stanford University, Stanford, CA 94305). This and other centers will assist organizations and individuals to develop projects in community-based health promotion in the following five areas: prevention of injuries, adolescent pregnancy, cardiovascular disease, cancer, and substance abuse.

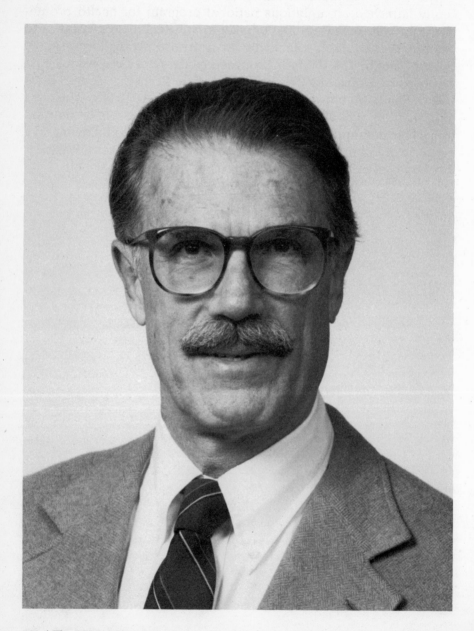

ABOUT THE AUTHOR

D r. John W. Farquhar, Director of the Stanford Center for Research in Disease Prevention, was born and raised in Winnipeg, Canada. He was graduated from the University of California, Berkeley, and earned his M.D. degree at the University of California, San Francisco, where he was awarded the prestigious Gold Headed Cane. A cardiologist, Dr. Farquhar joined the Stanford medical faculty in 1961 following four years at Rockefeller University in New York City. In 1968 he was visiting professor at the London School of Hygiene and Tropical Medicine, where he worked on the development of new methods in the study of cardiovascular epidemiology. He returned to Stanford in 1969 and established the Stanford Heart Disease Prevention Program in 1971. This multidisciplinary group at the Stanford Medical School was expanded into the Center for Research in Disease Prevention in 1984. The Center emphasis is on community-based, self-help approaches to the prevention and control of chronic diseases, substance abuse (including alcohol and tobacco), and injury and death by accident. Recently, the Center joined with the Kaiser Family Foundation to establish a pilot program for health promotion resource centers in the Western states.

In 1983 Dr. Farquhar was honored with the James D. Bruce Memorial Award by the American College of Physicians in recognition of distinguished achievement in preventive medicine. In addition to his teaching and research activities at Stanford, he is active in the World Health Organization of the United Nations and is a member of the Institute of Medicine of the National Academy of Sciences.

CREDITS

Sources for figures and tables appearing throughout the book are listed below.

Figure 1-1   Redrawn from R. Golubjatnikov, T. Paskey, and S. L. Inhorn, "Serum Cholesterol Levels of Mexican and Wisconsin School Children," *American Journal of Epidemiology*, vol. 96, 1972, p. 38.

Figure 1-2   Redrawn from Fig. 56, *Coronary Heart Disease in Seven Countries*, Ancel Keys, ed., American Heart Association Monograph No. 29, 1970, p. 191. Reproduced by permission of the American Heart Association, Inc.

Figure 1-3   Henry Blackburn, "Coronary Risk Factors: How to Evaluate and Manage Them," *European Journal of Cardiology*, 1975, 2/3, p. 251.

Table 1-1   The National Center for Health Statistics, Washington, DC.

Figure 1-4   H. A. Kahn, "The Dorn Study of Smoking and Mortality Among U.S. Veterans," Bethesda, Maryland: National Cancer Institute Monograph No. 19, January 1966, pp. 36-44.

Figure 1-5   Risk levels were calculated from an equation given in J. Truett, J. Cornfield, and W. Kannel, "Multivariate Analysis of the Risk of Coronary Heart Disease in Framingham," *Journal of Chronic Disease*, vol. 20, 1967, p. 511.

Figure 2-1   Photographs originally appeared in M. L. Armstrong, E. D. Warner, and W. E. Connor, "Regression of Coronary Atheromatosis in Rhesus Monkeys," *Circulation Research*, 1970, p. 68. Reproduced by permission of the American Heart Association, Inc.

Figure 6-1   *Dietary Goals for the United States*, 2nd ed., December 1977, p. 12. Select Committee on Nutrition and Human Needs, U.S. Senate.

INDEX

Action plans, 37, 49-53; exercise, 92-96; nutrition, 120-139; smoking cessation, 164, 168-178; stress management, 56, 64-77; weight control, 143, 150-157

Adrenalin, 56

Advertising: food, 23-24, 111; tobacco, 24-25, 36, 183-184

Aerobic exercise, 81-90 passim; program for, 93-94, 98-99

Aerobic Way, The (Cooper), 93

Africa, 110

African cuisine, northern, 109

Age-Grouped Running Program, 91

Aging, 11-12; and blood pressure, 8; and weight, 145-146, 147

Air pollution, 20

Alcohol control, 108, 123, 125, 131, 135, 136, 139; and weight control, 123

Amateur Athletic Union, 91

American Cancer Society, 167, 184

American Heart Association, 105, 112, 121, 184

American Heart Association Cookbook, The, 128

American Lung Association, 184

Americas, 110. *See also* North America

Amino acids, 109

Andes, Ecuadorian: longevity in, 11-12

Angina pectoris, 11

Antioxidants: anti-cancer benefits of, 108

Armstrong, Marc, 28

Arthritis, 86, 141

Asia, 110

Atherosclerosis, 3, 6, 10-11, 22, 56, 82, 106, 163; prevention of, 30, 32, 82-83; reversible, 28-30, 106

Australia, 109

Automation, 25

Bandura, Albert, 36

Becker, Marion, 124

Behavior modification, 35, 36-37. *See also* Self-directed change

Behavior-pattern awareness, 37, 46-49; and exercise, 92; and nutrition, 118-120; and smoking, 164, 167-168; and stress, 56, 60-64, 71; and weight, 143, 147-150

Belgium, 30, 104

Beta carotene: anti-cancer benefit of, 108

Bicycle Manufacturers Association of America, 32-33

Bicycling, 32-33, 81-89 passim, 93, 98

Biofeedback, 67

Birth control pills: risks of, 40

Blackburn, Henry, 15, 105

Blankenhorn, David, 30

Blood cholesterol, *see* Cholesterol

Blood pressure, high, 37, 130; and aging, 8; and cultural factors, 8-9, 102-104; and exercise, 80, 86, 87; and heart disease, 5, 15, 16, 40; measuring, 39-40, 86; as risk factor, 83, 99, 116; salt intake and, 6-7, 8, 9, 83, 86, 102-104, 112; and stress, 15-16; and weight control, 7, 8, 141, 145, 153, 161

Blood sugar level, 115, 120, 152

Breakfast, 119, 127-128

Breast cancer: diet and, 4, 19, 40, 108, 138

Breast-feeding, 160

Brody, Jane, 124

Bronchitis, winter, 20

Caffeine control, 122-125, 129, 130, 134, 138

Calcium, 4, 22, 110, 111, 130

California Dairy Association, 22

Calisthenics, 84

Caloric density, 113-115, 118, 120, 123, 130-139 passim; and weight control, 153-156, 160

Calories, 8, 15, 25, 37, 80, 146, 153; carbohydrate, 107; fat, 105, 107, 109; sugar, 106, 107

Cancer: deaths from, 4, 14, 19; and diet, 4, 19, 21, 40, 99, 107-109, 111, 121, 137, 138, 182-183; prevention of, 4, 80, 108-109; and smoking, 4, 13-14, 26, 40, 163

Carbohydrates, 24, 124; caloric density of, 115; complex, 107, 120, 123, 134, 137, 138; refined (see Sugar intake); and weight control, 107, 137

Cardiovascular disease: deaths from, 4, 11, 12, 20, 21, 30, 32, 82; and diet, 23, 101, 106, 111, 116, 121, 133, 138; prevention of, 3-4, 10, 12, 21, 55, 79-81, 82, 99, 105, 116, 141; risk factors in, 12, 15-17, 30, 37-38, 40, 53, 55, 86, 87, 94, 99, 145; and sedentary living, 81, 83; and smoking, 163, 167-168, 181. See also Heart disease; Strokes

Carnegie Foundation, 184

Caucasus, Soviet: longevity in, 11-12

Central American cuisine, 109

Cereal grains, 109, 111, 115, 120; and cancer prevention, 108-109

Chewing gum, nicotine-containing, 164, 177

Chewing tobacco, 25, 184

Children: cholesterol levels of, 5-6; eating habits of, 4-7, 8, 23, 104, 109-110, 146; and exercise, 79; obesity prevention in, 160; smoking among, 32, 36

Cholesterol, 3, 11, 22, 23, 37, 104-106, 116, 142; and cultural factors, 5-6, 8, 9-10, 105, 112; and early eating habits, 4-7, 8; and exercise, 80, 82; and heart disease, 9-10, 16, 29-30, 40, 105; measuring levels of, 39-40, 86; and stress, 15, 56; reducing, 115, 118, 120, 121, 124, 133-134, 138, 141, 145; as risk factor, 37, 83, 94, 99; and weight control, 142, 153-154, 161

Chronic disease: risk factors in, 37-38, 86, 87, 99, 116

Cigarette smoking, see Smoking

Closing Circle, The (Commoner), 26

Colon cancer: diet and, 4, 19, 40, 108, 138

Commitment, see Confidence and commitment

Commoner, Barry, 26

Complete Aerobic Program (Cooper), 93

Complete Walker, The (Fletcher), 91

Confidence and commitment, 37, 42, 45-46; in exercise, 87, 92; in nutrition, 117-118; in smoking cessation, 164, 167; in stress management, 56, 60, 70, 71; in weight control, 143, 147, 160

Connor, Sonja, 128

Connor, William, 28, 112, 128

Consensus conferences, 28

Conservatism, scientific, 25-28, 112

Constipation: decrease in, 138

Convenience foods, 24, 120

Cooper, Kenneth, 93

Crapo, Lawrence, 11

Cultural factors: an blood pressure, 8-9, 102-104; and cholesterol levels, 5-6, 9-10, 105, 112; and heart disease, 9-10, 12; and ill health, 36, 112, 183; and milk myth, 109-110; and protein myth, 109, 112; and rich-food fixation, 111, 112; and sedentary living, 80

Dahl, Lewis, 104

Dairy consumption, 104, 105; changes in, 33, 112, 121, 126, 133, 134, 138; excessive, 4, 6, 9, 22, 32, 83, 109, 112; and milk myth, 109, 111

and smoking, 3, 14, 26, 32, 40, 163; surgery for, 21. *See also* Cardiovascular disease

Hemorrhoids: decrease in, 138

Herodotus, 183

Himalayas: longevity in, 11-12

Holland, 30

Hutchins, Robert, 42

Hypoglycemia, 120

Identification of problems, 37-45; exercise, 87-91; nutrition, 116; smoking, 164-167; stress, 56, 57-60, 71; weight, 143, 144-147

Imagery training, 67-68, 94, 95, 99, 128, 170

Immigrants, U.S.: heart disease among, 10; weight gain among, 146

India, 110

Indian cuisine, 133

Indoles: anti-cancer benefit of, 108

Insulin, 106, 120

Isotonic exercise, 85

Jane Brody's Good Food Book, 124

Japanese: blood pressure levels of, 103; cholesterol levels of, 9, 105; weight of, 146

Jogging, 81, 85, 87, 93, 96

Johnson, John, 110

Joy of Cooking, The (Rombauer and Becker), 124

Junk foods, 112

Kaiser Family Foundation, 184

Kannel, William, 16

Kellog Foundation, 184

Ketosis, 142

Keys, Ancel, 9, 105

Koreans: cholesterol levels of, 9

Kretchmer, Norman, 110

Lactate, 56

Lactose assimilation: differences in, 110-111

"Lactose Malabsorption: Its Biology and History" (Johnson, Kretchmer, and Simoons), 110

Lappé, Frances Moore, 116, 124

Latin American cuisine, 109

Leaf, Alexander, 11

Legumes, 115, 120, 137

Life expectancy, 11-12, 19, 28

Life-style, 4; changes in, 30, 32, 36. *See also* Sedentary living; Self-directed change

Lipids, *see* Cholesterol; Triglycerides

Lipoproteins, 82, 106

Liquid protein diet: hazards of, 142

London: winter bronchitis in, 20

Longevity, 11-12, 19, 28

Lunch, 119, 120, 128

Lung cancer: smoking and, 4, 13-14, 26, 40, 163

Lung disease, 4, 13, 20, 163. *See also* Lung cancer

Luthe, W., 64

McDonald's restaurant chain, 24

McGinnis, J. Michael, 28

Mahoney, Kathryn, 39, 43

Mahoney, Michael, 39, 43

Maintenance of changes, 53; exercise, 96-99; nutrition, 131-132, 136-137, 139; smoking cessation, 164, 178-181; stress management, 56, 77; weight control, 143, 157-160

Man Adapting (Dubos), 19

Mayer, Jean, 24, 53

Meal spacing, 119-120

Meat consumption, 104, 105, 111, 160; decline in, 33, 112; excessive, 4, 6, 9, 22, 32, 83, 109, 112; reducing, 115, 121, 128, 133, 134

Medical Economics (journal), 32

Mediterranean cuisine, 109, 124, 133, 138

Meichenbaum, Donald, 71

Mental illness, 64

Mental relaxation, 66-71, 74, 77, 136, 158, 171

Merrill, John, 91

Metabolism, 146

Mexican children: cholesterol levels of, 5-6

Mexican cuisine, 133

Middle Eastern cuisine, 109, 124, 133

Milk, whole: myth about, 109-111; vs. nonfat and low-fat, 33, 110-111, 121, 126. *See also* Dairy consumption

Muscles: loss of, 14; relaxation of, 64-71, 74, 77, 131, 136, 158, 171, 176; tightness of, 56

National Cancer Institute, 108, 115
National Geographic (magazine), 11
National Institutes of Health, 28, 184
National Research Council, 101, 108
New Aerobics, The (Cooper), 93
New American Diet, The (Connor and Connor), 128
New Zealand, 109
Nicorette (chewing gum), 117
1984 (Orwell), 36
Noradrenalin, 56
Normality: false attribution of, 15-16, 103, 143
North America, 109
Norway, 30
Nutrition: and cancer, 4, 19, 21, 40, 99, 101, 107-109, 111, 137, 138, 182-183; education about, 23-24, 102, 183, 184; influence of advertising on, 23-24, 111; and program of alternative food pattern, 102, 113-139; as risk factor, 99. *See also* Eating habits; Overweight; Weight control

Obesity, 15, 37, 80, 101, 106, 111, 138, 141; in children, 160. *See also* Overweight; Weight control
Oils, *see* Fat intake; Vegetable fats and oils
Orwell, George, 36
Osteoarthritis, 141
Osteoporosis: prevention of, 80, 99
Overeaters Anonymous, 147
Overweight, 7-8, 9, 14-15, 25, 37, 41, 80, 143; assessing, 39, 144-145; and heart disease, 40; myths about, 145-147; as risk factor, 99, 141, 145; smoking cessation and, 172, 181. *See also* Obesity; Weight control

Paffenbarger, Ralph, 81
Page, Lot, 8
Permanent Weight Control (Mahoney and Mahoney), 39, 43
Peto, Richard, 108
Pfaffman, Carl, 106

Phosphate, 111
Physician-patient relationship, 35-36
Political action, 26-28, 184-185
Positive thinking, 43-45, 46, 72, 91, 99, 150, 158, 165, 170
Potassium, 142
Prevention, 11, 28, 185; barriers to, 25, 26-27, 28; of cardiovascular disease, 3-4, 10, 12, 21, 55, 79-81, 82, 99, 105, 116, 141; education for, 22, 26
Prevention '84/85 (government report), 28
Price, Virginia, 58
Processed foods, 24, 111
Progesterone, 40
Prospects for a Healthier America (government report), 28
Protein consumption, 22-23, 107, 110, 115, 120, 137; of children, 4; myth about, 109, 112; and weight control, 107, 142
Public health, 27-28, 184-185
Pulse rate: and exercise, 81, 85; and stress, 56, 81

Recipes for a Small Planet (Ewald), 124
Record keeping, 45, 48-49; exercise, 88, 92, 94; nutrition, 113, 118; smoking cessation, 168; stress management, 61-64, 71, 72, 75-76; weight control, 148-150
Rectal cancer: and diet, 4, 108, 138
Reid, Donald, 26
Relaxation, muscle and mental, 64-71, 74, 77, 131, 136, 158, 171, 176
Relaxation tapes, 67-68
Research: and prevention, 26-27
Restaurants, 105, 132; fast-food, 24, 104, 111-112
Rogers, Will, 28
Rombauer, Irma, 124
Rosenman, Ray, 58
Running, 81, 83, 87, 89
Rynearson, Edward, 145

Salt intake, 24, 154; and blood pressure, 6-7, 8, 9, 83, 86, 102-104, 112; and cardiovascular disease, 23, 83; reducing, 94, 108, 115-138 passim
Saturated fats, *see* Fat intake
Schultz, V. H., 64

Scientific conservatism, 25-28, 112
Sedentary living, 79; and cardio-
vascular disease, 81, 83; and weight
gain, 14-15, 25, 37, 41, 80, 145-146,
157, 160
Self-contracts, 42; exercise, 87, 91,
93-94; nutrition, 127-128, 132; smok-
ing cessation, 173, 177; stress man-
agement, 49-50, 60, 70, 74, 76; weight
control, 147, 154-155, 160
Self-directed change: achieving, 36-53,
164
Self-responsibility, 33, 35-36
Self-reward, 50-51, 72-74, 77, 95-96,
132, 136, 139, 158
"Seven Country Coronary Disease
Study" (Keys and Blackburn), 105
Skiing, 81
Sierra Club, 91
Snacks, 6, 111-112, 120, 132; and
weight gain, 7, 152, 153, 181
Simoons, Frederick, 110
Sleep disorders, 141
Smoking, 12, 32, 36, 37; and advertising, 24-25, 36, 183-184; decline in, 32;
and heart disease, 3, 14, 26, 32, 40,
163; impact on health, 4, 163; and
lung cancer, 4, 13-14, 26, 40; program
for quitting, 51, 53, 55, 56, 80,
163-181; as risk factor, 37, 83; and
weight gain on quitting, 172, 181
Social environment, 46-48, 183
Social support, 49, 50; exercise, 92, 96;
nutrition, 136, 137-138; smoking cessation, 167, 172, 176, 178, 179, 181;
stress management, 69-70, 72; weight
control, 158
Sodium, 104, 130, 160. See also Salt
intake
Solomon Islanders: blood pressure levels of, 103-104; effects of acculturation among, 8-9
South Pacific, 110
Soviet Caucasus: longevity in, 11-12
Stanford Center for Research in Disease Prevention, 40, 51, 55, 58, 61,
64, 66, 71, 104, 164, 168-169
Stanford Medical School, 30
Starch, 106, 107, 115
Starvation diets, 142, 151
Stress, 4, 37, 112; coping with, 43, 46,
53, 55-77, 80, 94, 145, 165, 184; effects

on health, 15, 56; and physiological
changes, 56; as risk factor, 55
Strokes, 3, 21, 182; death from, 4, 11,
12, 20; decrease in rate of, 12, 21;
prevention of, 3, 12, 21, 56; risk
factors in, 40-41, 56. See also Cardiovascular disease
Sugar intake, 24, 106-107, 118, 160; and
cardiovascular disease, 23, 32, 106;
and diabetes, 106, 111; excessive, 7,
8, 37, 106, 111, 112; reducing, 115,
116, 120-126 passim, 133-134, 135,
137, 138
Surgeon General's report: of 1964, 26,
32; of 1979, 27-28
Surgery, 141; heart, 21
Sweden, 12
Swim Masters Program, 91
Swimming, 81, 83, 86, 87, 91, 93

Tapes, relaxation, 67-68
Tarlov, Alvin, 28
Tennis, 83, 87, 93
Tension, see Stress
Thoresen, Carl, 37, 43
Thyroid deficiency, 145
Tobacco, smokeless, 25. See also
Smoking
Tooth decay, 106, 138
TOPS (Take Off Pounds Sensibly), 33,
147
Triglycerides, 82, 106, 161
Twain, Mark, 53
Type A behavior, 58, 59, 89
Type A Behavior and Your Heart (Fried-
man and Rosenman), 58

U.S. Department of Health and Human
Services, 28
U.S. Nutrition Policies in the Seventies
(Mayer), 24
U.S. Public Health Service, 24, 184;
Office of Disease Prevention and
Health Promotion, 28

Vegetable fats and oils, 23, 105
Vegetables, 105, 109, 111, 116, 120;
caloric density of, 115; and cancer
prevention, 108-109; as protein
source, 109, 120, 134, 137